CLINICAL GASTROENTEROLOGY

Series Editor
George Y. Wu
University of Connecticut Health Center
Farmington, CT, USA

More information about this series at http://www.springer.com/series/7672

Michael L. Schilsky
Editor

Management of Wilson Disease

A Pocket Guide

Humana Press

Editor
Michael L. Schilsky
Yale New Haven
Transplantation Center
Yale University
New Haven, CT
USA

ISSN 2197-7399 ISSN 2197-7704 (electronic)
Clinical Gastroenterology
ISBN 978-3-319-91526-5 ISBN 978-3-319-91527-2 (eBook)
https://doi.org/10.1007/978-3-319-91527-2

Library of Congress Control Number: 2018952074

Printed on acid-free paper

This Humana Press imprint is published by the registered company Springer Nature Switzerland AG
The registered company address is: Gewerbestrasse 11, 6330 Cham, Switzerland

Preface

The cornerstone of achieving best care and maximizing outcome for disease management is the partnership between health care provider and patient. This "Handbook" was therefore targeted to primary physicians to help them understand more about the underlying physiology, diagnosis, and treatment of the rare disorder, Wilson disease. We have focused the subjects included on what we consider relevant care issues for patients. Patients may also benefit from reading this book and discussing specific subject matter with their caregivers. Whether read by the primary care or other treating health care provider or patient, our aim is to stimulate conversation between patient and their caregivers in order for them to achieve the individualization of care they need, recognizing that many patients have different expression of their disease and differing degrees of disability. We therefore have tasked our authors to cover important topics with an eye toward making the subject matter both informative and practical. I am grateful for the time and effort of the many experts from the Center of Excellence for Wilson Disease at Yale and for my colleagues outside of our institution who have graciously shared their expertise to make this very readable and useful guide to Wilson disease. As editor and contributing author, I must also acknowledge my debt of gratitude to my mentor, the late Professor Irmin Sternlieb, who shared his passion for learning and care of patients with me, and to the many patients with Wilson disease from whom

I continue to learn and share life experiences. We hope you find this “Handbook” useful and that it helps foster better care partnerships between patient and health care providers and thereby improve quality of life and outcomes for patients with Wilson disease.

New Haven, CT, USA Michael L. Schilsky

Contents

Contributors

Nigel S. Bamford Department of Neurology, Yale University, New Haven, CT, USA

Department of Pediatrics, Yale University, New Haven, CT, USA

Department of Cellular and Molecular Physiology, Yale University, New Haven, CT, USA

Michelle Camarata Department of Gastroenterology and Hepatology, Royal Surrey County Hospital, Guildford, Surrey, UK

Department of Clinical and Experimental Medicine, University of Surrey, Guildford, Surrey, UK

Department of Surgery, Section of Transplant and Immunology, Yale School of Medicine, New Haven, CT, USA

Regino P. Gonzalez-Peralta Division of Pediatric Gastroenterology, Hepatology and Liver Transplantation, Florida Hospital for Children, Orlando, FL, USA

Mary L. Graper Wilson Disease Association, New York, NY, USA

Lenore Hammers Yale New Haven Transplantation Center, Liver Transplant Program, New Haven, CT, USA

Claire Kelly Department of Gastroenterology and Hepatology, Royal Surrey County Hospital, Surrey, UK

Department of Clinical and Experimental Medicine, University of Surrey, Surrey, UK

Tamir Miloh Pediatric Hepatology and Liver Transplant Medicine, Texas Children's Hospital, Houston, TX, USA

Baylor College of Medicine, Houston, TX, USA

Sahil Munjal Yale University School of Medicine, New Haven, CT, USA

Marinos Pericleous Department of Gastroenterology and Hepatology, Royal Surrey County Hospital, Surrey, UK

Department of Clinical and Experimental Medicine, University of Surrey, Surrey, UK

Anne Marie Rivard Department of Food and Nutrition, Yale New Haven Hospital, New Haven, CT, USA

Daphne Robakis Department of Neurology, Yale University, New Haven, CT, USA

Michael L. Schilsky Division of Digestive Diseases and Transplant and Immunology, Departments of Medicine and Surgery, Yale University, New Haven, CT, USA

Uyen To Division of Digestive Diseases, Department of Medicine, Yale University, New Haven, CT, USA

Ricarda Tomlin Yale University, School of Medicine, Department of Surgery/Transplant, New Haven, CT, USA

Ana Vives-Rodriguez Department of Neurology, Yale University, New Haven, CT, USA

Paula C. Zimbrean Department of Psychiatry, Yale University School of Medicine, New Haven, CT, USA

Chapter 1
Introduction to Copper Metabolism and Wilson Disease

Uyen To and Michael L. Schilsky

Introduction

Copper is an essential trace element that is important for proper growth and development [1]. It belongs to a class of trace elements known as essential elements because we require them for critical body functions and need to obtain them from our environment through our diets. A primary function of copper in the body is in metabolic reactions where it functions as an oxidizing agent [5]. Copper can participate in these reactions by changing its oxidation state. Some enzymes contain several copper atoms per molecule of protein and are known as multi-copper oxidases. These include the proteins ceruloplasmin,

U. To
Division of Digestive Diseases, Department of Medicine, Yale University, New Haven, CT, USA
e-mail: uyen.to@yale.edu

M. L. Schilsky (✉)
Division of Digestive Diseases and Transplant and Immunology, Departments of Medicine and Surgery, Yale University, New Haven, CT, USA
e-mail: michael.schilsky@yale.edu

M. L. Schilsky (ed.), *Management of Wilson Disease*, Clinical Gastroenterology, https://doi.org/10.1007/978-3-319-91527-2_1

hephaestin, and zyklopen that can take advantage of the change in oxidation state of copper to help with iron metabolism, allowing reduction of iron from Fe^{2+} to Fe^{3+} to facilitate iron transport and absorption [5]. Copper is also important for the function of lysyl oxidase, an enzyme that functions in cross-linking collagen and elastin in connective tissue in the muscle, bone, heart, and blood vessels [6]. Copper is incorporated into enzymes that act as antioxidants such as superoxide dismutase that remove damaging free radicals, and can also regulate expression of certain genes, based on the cellular level of oxidative stress [7]. It is also an important cofactor for blood cell formation and neurotransmitter synthesis [2]. Hence, deficiencies in copper can lead to low blood counts, infections, poor bone health, and neurologic symptoms [3].

In an average diet, daily dietary intake of copper is approximately 2–5 mg per day with a recommended minimum intake of 0.9 mg per day in adults [1, 8]. In infants and children, the recommended intake is approximately 0.2–0.7 mg/day [8]. When ingested, cells in the gut located in the duodenum and proximal small intestine absorb approximately 50% of dietary copper [1]. The copper then enters the portal venous system and is transported mostly bound to the protein albumin and some other peptides from which it is absorbed by the liver. In the liver, a portion of it is used for metabolic functions and incorporation into proteins, some is stored in the cells, some is released into the circulation, and the remaining copper not needed for metabolism is excreted into bile [9]. Most excess dietary copper is excreted into bile, but unlike other bile content such as bile acids that are reabsorbed, copper that enters bile is excreted into the stool. Excretion of copper by the kidneys that extract copper from the circulation is normally a minor pathway (<30 mg per day) [9]. The balance of copper in the body is achieved through regulation of uptake from the small intestine and excretion into the bile [10] (Fig. 1.1). Processes that impair the balance of copper uptake and excretion can lead to the toxic accumulation of copper in organs, first in the liver and then in the brain, kidney, retina, and other organs [1, 10].

The liver is central to copper metabolism, and therefore it is important to understand its normal function and potential dysfunction following injury. The liver performs approxi-

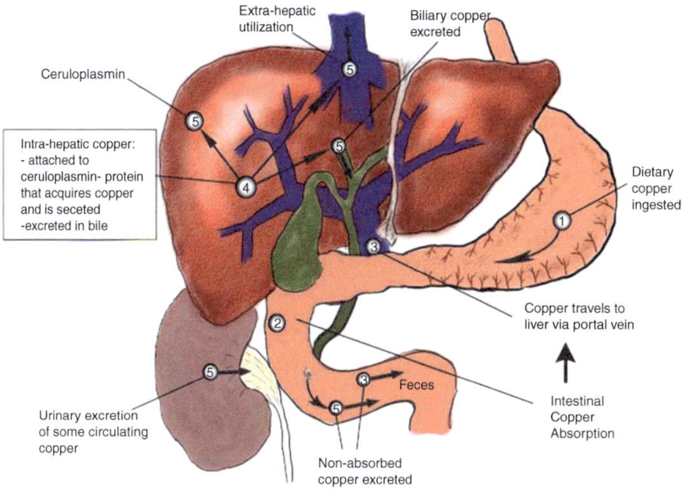

FIGURE. 1.1 Copper absorption in the body. Daily dietary intake of copper is approximately 2–5 mg per day. Approximately 50% of copper absorption occurs in the cells in the gut located in the duodenum and proximal small intestine. The copper then enters the portal venous system and is transported to the liver mostly bound to the protein albumin. In the liver, a portion of transported copper is used for metabolic functions and incorporation into proteins. Some of the copper is stored in the cells, some released into the circulation, and the remaining copper (not needed for metabolism) is excreted into bile. In normal individuals, excess dietary copper is ultimately excreted into bile, and excretion of copper by the kidneys is normally a minor pathway

mately 500 functions in the human body [11]. It synthesizes a number of biologically important molecules including fats, carbohydrates, and amino acids and metabolizes a broad range of molecules [11]. The liver also facilitates the digestion and storage of nutrients [11]. The liver has a dual blood supply and is fed predominantly from the hepatic portal vein (which brings blood rich with nutrients from the intestine and blood from the spleen) and to a lesser extent also receives blood supply from the supply hepatic artery [11]. The primary liver cells known as hepatocytes also produce and export bile into the bile canaliculus that leads to the biliary tracts that form the larger bile ducts, bringing the bile to the intestine [11].

Injury to the liver can occur immediatel (acutely) or from chronic inflammation [11]. In response to chronic injury, specialized cells in the liver called hepatic stellate cells become activated and induce scarring through the secretion of collagen, which is known as fibrosis. Over time, extensive and advancing fibrosis can lead to cirrhosis with its complications of changes in blood supply known as portal hypertension. The clinical manifestations of portal hypertension and the complications that ensue in patients are discussed in a later chapter.

Cellular Mechanisms of Copper Transport

While general mechanisms for copper transport outside the liver are not affected in WD, it is useful to have a good understanding of copper transport to better understand overall copper metabolism. This process is reviewed in Fig. 1.2. To facilitate transport, copper in the intestinal lumen is initially changed in its oxidation state and reduced from Cu^{2+} to Cu^{1+} by an enzyme called metalloreductase on the cell membrane of a small intestine cell called an enterocyte [12]. Copper is then transported into the cell by a membrane protein called CTR1 that is expressed in all human tissues and which is abundant in the liver. Human cells have

FIGURE. 1.2 Copper metabolism in the liver cell. Copper bound to albumin is transported from the blood into the liver cell by a membrane protein called CTR1. After copper uptake into the cell, carrier proteins known as metallochaperones shuttle copper to enzymes and other metal ion transporters. The liver utilizes the copper for metabolic needs and the hepatocyte incorporates it into important enzymes, such as ceruloplasmin, and stores it bound to small molecules like metallothionein that keep it from injuring other cell components. ATP7B is usually located in cells in an organelle known as the trans-Golgi network in normal conditions and functions here to transport copper for incorporation into ceruloplasmin. However, when copper levels are high, ATP7B transports copper into vesicles that move to the apical portion of the cell membrane to release their contents that includes copper into bile

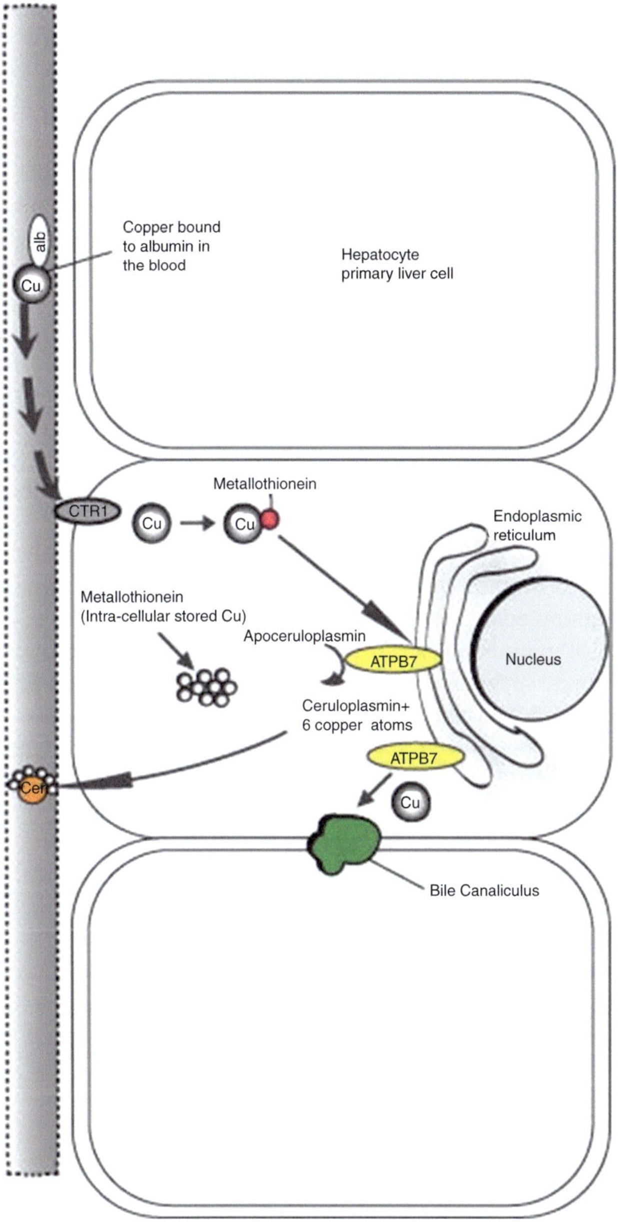
alb
Cu
Copper bound to albumin in the blood
Hepatocyte primary liver cell
Metallothionein
CTR1
Cu
Cu
Endoplasmic reticulum
Metallothionein (Intra-cellular stored Cu)
Apoceruloplasmin
ATPB7
Nucleus
Ceruloplasmin+ 6 copper atoms
ATPB7
Cer
Cu
Bile Canaliculus

adapted to their environment by clever mechanisms for changing the amount of this copper transporter on the surface of cells. CTR1 normally resides in small envelopes called vesicles within cells, and moves to the cell surface when copper levels are low to facilitate new copper uptake, but this transporter is degraded in states of copper abundance to reduce new transport into cells [13].

After copper uptake into cells, a carrier protein called a metallochaperone shuttles copper to enzymes and other metal ion transporters, including ATP7A (the Menkes disease gene protein) and ATP7B (the WD gene protein) [14]. Both of these proteins are important for maintaining copper balance, as they transport copper to other compartments of the cell for incorporation into copper-dependent enzymes and for export to the bloodstream [15]. ATP7A is present in many tissues, but ATP7B is predominantly expressed in primary liver cells or hepatocytes and, to a lesser degree, in the kidney, brain, heart, cornea, erythrocytes, joints, and lungs [15].

ATP7A exports the absorbed copper from enterocytes into the bloodstream. The copper then travels bound to albumin or the amino acid histidine to the liver. The liver utilizes the copper for metabolic needs and incorporates it into important enzymes, such as ceruloplasmin, superoxide dismutase, and cytochrome proteins, and stores it bound to molecules like metallothionein that keep it from injuring other cell components. Both ATP7A and ATP7B proteins can relocate within cells to facilitate copper export or import depending on the abundance or scarcity of copper [16]. ATP7B is usually located in cells in an organelle known as the trans-Golgi network in normal conditions and functions here to transport copper for incorporation into ceruloplasmin. However, when copper levels are high, ATP7B transports copper into vesicles that move to the apical portion of the cell membrane to release their contents that includes copper for excretion into bile [17].

Wilson Disease

Wilson disease (WD) is a rare autosomal recessive disorder of copper metabolism that affects multiple organ systems throughout the body [1]. The World Health Organization estimates the global prevalence of WD as between 1 in 10,000 and 1 in 30,000 people [18]. WD was initially described in 1912 by the American-born but British-trained neurologist, Sir Samuel Alexander Kinnier Wilson, who identified characteristic changes in the brain and liver and linked the neurologic disease to cirrhosis of the liver [19]. However, it was neuropathologist John Nathaniel Cumings who made the link between copper accumulation in the liver and the brain as the etiology of WD [20]. It was not until 1993 that three different groups reported on the discovery of the WD gene and identified the defect as affecting the copper-transporting protein ATP7B, located on chromosome 13q14 [21–23].

WD results from mutations or defective function of the ATP7B protein [24]. Many different specific variants of the *ATP7B* gene have been identified, including single or multiple missense mutations, frameshift deletions, splice site mutations, or truncating mutations, among others [25]. Certain variants are more common in specific populations, likely reflecting a founder effect. There are over 500 disease-causing mutations of *ATP7B* that have been recorded for the ATP7B gene. The most common mutations are H1069Q in exon 14, commonly seen in patients of European descent, and the R778L mutation in Asian populations. We all have two copies of our genes on our chromosomes. To have WD a patient needs to have a mutation of both copies of the gene. Given the wide range of genetic backgrounds in populations, most individuals with WD carry two different mutations, one on each allele (with one copy of the gene on each) of chromosome 13 [26, 27]. More information on ATP7B is discussed in the next chapter that focuses on WD diagnosis.

Abnormal Copper Metabolism and Injury in Wilson Disease

Lack of the ATP7B protein or its dysfunction leads to toxic copper accumulation within hepatocytes due to an inability to export the copper into bile [16]. The mechanism of copper-induced injury cellular is the generation of reactive oxygen species [30]. In the presence of reducing agents, Cu^{2+} is reduced to Cu^{1+} and then is reoxidized via an oxygen molecule, thus generating an O_2 radical from oxygen and OH radical from H_2O_2 [7, 30]. These hydroxyl radicals can cause DNA oxidation and breaks and membrane lipid peroxidative damage, directly inhibit protein activity, impair mitochondrial function, and induce cell death by a mechanism called apoptosis (programmed cell death) via its inhibition of the antiapoptotic protein X-linked inhibitor of apoptosis (XIAP) [7, 30, 31] (Fig. 1.3). The oxidative damage produced by copper can then activate hepatic stellate cells within the liver to secrete collagen and produce scarring or fibrosis in the liver and, over time, this leads to cirrhosis. The degree of liver injury and timing of the disease are variable between patients. This is due not only to different degrees of ATP7B dysfunction in some patients but to many factors including the dietary intake of copper, an individual's antioxidant capacity, hormonal influences, and individual susceptibility to hepatic fibrosis [32, 33]. The natural course of the histology findings in the liver that is seen in WD is demonstrated in Fig. 1.4. Initially copper accumulation in the liver can

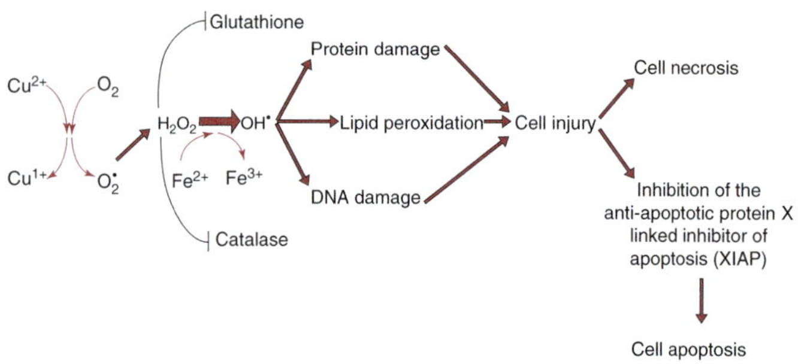

FIGURE. 1.3 Copper-induced cell injury. The mechanism of copper-induced injury cellular is the generation of reactive oxygen species. In the presence of reducing agents, Cu^{2+} is reduced to Cu^{1+} and then is reoxidized via an oxygen molecule, thus generating an O_2 radical from oxygen and OH radical from H_2O_2. These hydroxyl radicals can cause DNA oxidation and breaks and membrane lipid peroxidative damage and directly inhibit protein synthesis and activity. Depending on the conditions and cell type, it can induce cell death by "necrosis" or "apoptosis" (*aka* programmed cell death)

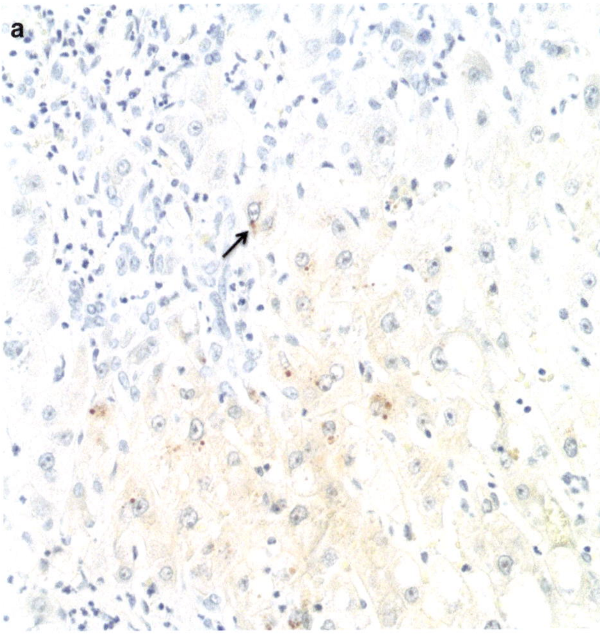

FIGURE. 1.4 (**a**) On liver biopsy, copper (arrow pointing at red pigment) can be stained, detected, and quantified in liver cells. (Micrographs courtesy of Dr. Romulo Celli, used with permission). (**b**) Inflammation (black arrow shows areas of dense inflammatory cells that appear as denser purple dots on the micrograph) and focal Mallory's hyaline (blue arrow indicating aggregates of the cell "skeleton" that are in the cell that result from liver cell injury appearing as more dense pink areas) are typically seen in earlier stage of the disease. (Micrographs courtesy of Dr. Romulo Celli, used with permission). (**c**) Inflammation and scarring (fibrosis) occurring from the chronic inflammation is seen here (black arrow). Large droplets of fat (steatosis) can also be seen early on in Wilson disease. (seen as clear areas in cells, blue arrow). (*Micrographs courtesy of Dr. Romulo Celli, used with permission*). (**d**) Cirrhotic liver as end stage of Wilson disease. Here we see a regenerative nodule that is surrounded by a band of fibrosis. (black arrow). (*Micrographs courtesy of Dr. Romulo Celli, used with permission*)

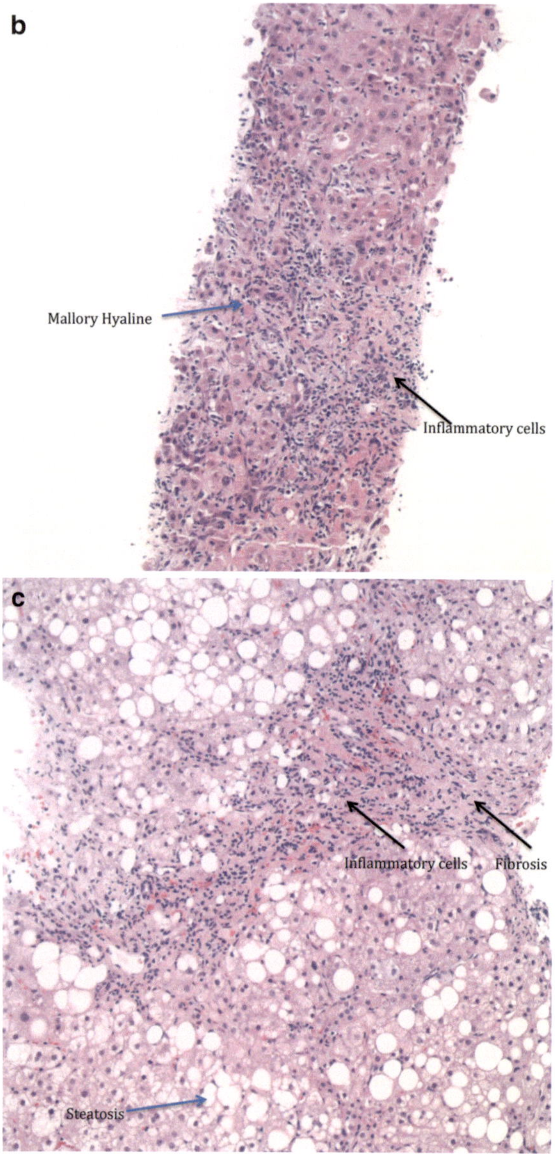

FIGURE. 1.4 (continued)

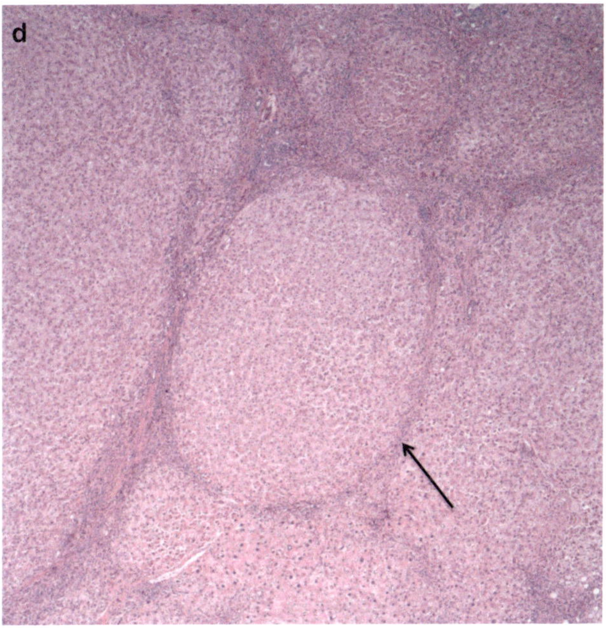

FIGURE. 1.4 (continued)

present with moderate steatosis (fat in the liver cells) and mild steatohepatitis(fat with associated inflammation). As the inflammation progresses, the steatosis can become more severe and fibrosis occurs, ultimately resulting in cirrhosis.

Lack of ATP7B transport function also leads to failure of copper incorporation into ceruloplasmin [15] in the trans-Golgi network of hepatocytes. Apoceruloplasmin (ceruloplasmin peptide without copper) has a shorter circulating half-life than holoceruloplasmin (with copper), and thus the apoprotein is cleared more rapidly, accounting for the low steady-state level of ceruloplasmin in the serum of most patients with WD [1].

Ceruloplasmin: A Marker of Wilson Disease and Copper Status

Ceruloplasmin is synthesized by hepatocytes in the liver and secreted from the liver into circulation as a copper-carrying protein. It is the major copper-containing protein in the blood [1]. It also functions mainly as a "ferroxidase" by assisting in iron absorption by reducing Fe2+ to Fe3+ within the enterocyte to allow it to be transported via a protein called ferroportin [5]. Interestingly, a mutation in the ceruloplasmin gene leading to complete loss of production of this protein, a disorder known as aceruloplasminemia, results in iron but not copper overload in the liver, brain, and pancreas [28]. Although ceruloplasmin is low in WD, iron overload does not contribute to the natural pathogenesis of the disease unless the patient also has a disorder of iron metabolism as well as WD [29]. Interestingly, overtreatment of WD can lead to a relative copper deficiency and further reduction of levels of ceruloplasmin with subsequent iron accumulation in liver cells that can be injurious. This is discussed in the chapter on treatment of WD.

Levels of ceruloplasmin can fluctuate in a normal individual, and cannot (in isolation) be reliably used as a single test in isolation for diagnosis of WD [1] (see section on diagnosis of WD). The serum non-ceruloplasmin-bound copper concentration can be used to monitor treatment of WD and is reviewed later in the section on treatment monitoring. The excretion of copper in the urine increases when there is excess copper in the circulation in untreated or poorly treated WD and is helpful for diagnosis and also for treatment monitoring.

When Copper Is in Excess

Beyond the liver, copper accumulation can also cause injury to cells within the brain. Although the mechanism is not entirely clear, copper injury in the brain results from an increase in brain copper and impaired copper homeostasis and repair mechanisms. In particular astrocytes in the brain are prone to copper injury. Normally metallothionein and glutathione in these cells binds, stores, and detoxifies metals including copper. In the presence of high amounts of copper, glutathione can become oxidized and this metallothionein-bound copper can become harmful as their oxidative by-products attack the binding sites of the metal-protein complex. Over time the copper accumulation then leads to cellular swelling and death. The other potential neurotoxicity of copper overload is copper's interference with the synthesis of the neurotransmitter dopamine, which along with injury to the basal ganglia may lead to the clinical findings of Parkinsonism seen in the disease [34, 35].

Summary and Conclusion

WD is caused by defects in the *ATP7B* gene that encodes a copper-transporting ATPase mainly expressed in liver cells. In WD, copper accumulates in the liver where it causes oxidative injury and cellular dysfunction and cell death, and the response to injury leads to progressive fibrosis and cirrhosis. Once the liver accumulates copper beyond its safe storage capacity, copper then accumulates in other organs, in particular in the brain, where it may cause injury and clinical disease. In the following chapters, we detail how the pathophysiology of defective copper metabolism in WD leads to clinical disease in children and adults. We discuss disease diagnosis, treatments, and monitoring of treatment for patients. Having a knowledge of the normal metabolism of the essential element copper and the changes that occur in WD helps us to better understand the natural history of the disease, its variability, and approaches to treatment and monitoring.

References

1. Roberts EA, Schilsky ML. American Association for Study of liver D. Diagnosis and treatment of Wilson disease: an update. Hepatology. 2008;47(6):2089–111.
2. Scheiber IF, Mercer JF, Dringen R. Metabolism and functions of copper in brain. Prog Neurobiol. 2014;116:33–57.
3. Lazarchick J. Update on anemia and neutropenia in copper deficiency. Curr Opin Hematol. 2012;19(1):58–60.
4. Pfeiffer R. Wilson's disease. Semin Neurol. 2007;27(2):123–32.
5. Pfeiffenberger J, Gotthardt DN, Herrmann T, et al. Iron metabolism and the role of HFE gene polymorphisms in Wilson disease. Liver Int. 2012;32(1):165–70.
6. Rucker RB, Kosonen T, Clegg MS, et al. Copper, lysyl oxidase, and extracellular matrix protein cross-linking. Am J Clin Nutr. 1998;67(5 Suppl):996S–1002S.
7. Halliwell B, JMC G. Role of free radicals and catalytic metal ions in human disease: an overview. Methods Enzymol. 1990;186:1–85.
8. (US) NAP. Dietary Reference Intakes for Vitamin A, Vitamin K, Arsenic, Boron, Chromium, Copper, Iodine, Iron, Manganese, Molybdenum, Nickel, Silicon, Vanadium, and Zinc. 2001.
9. Crampton RF, Matthews DM, Poisner R. Observations on the mechanism of absorption of copper by the small intestine. J Physiol. 1965;178(1):111–26.
10. Ferenci P. Pathophysiology and clinical features of Wilson disease. Metab Brain Dis. 2004;19(3/4):229–39.
11. Zakim D, Thomas DB. Hepatology: a textbook of liver disease. 4th ed; 2002.
12. Hassett R, Kosman DJ. Evidence for Cu(II) reduction as a component of copper uptake by Saccharomyces cerevisiae. J Biol Chem. 1995;270(1):128–34.
13. Lee J, Pena MM, Nose Y, Thiele DJ. Biochemical characterization of the human copper transporter Ctr1. J Biol Chem. 2002;277(6):4380–7.
14. Wernimont AK, Huffman DL, Lamb AL, O'Halloran TV, Rosenzweig AC. Structural basis for copper transfer by the

metallochaperone for the Menkes/Wilson disease proteins. Nat Struct Biol. 2000;7(9):766–71.
15. Lutsenko S, Barnes NL, Bartee MY, Dmitriev OY. Function and regulation of human copper-transporting ATPases. Physiol Rev. 2007;87(3):1011–46.
16. La Fontaine S, Mercer JF. Trafficking of the copper-ATPases, ATP7A and ATP7B: role in copper homeostasis. Arch Biochem Biophys. 2007;463(2):149–67.
17. Nyasae L, Bustos R, Braiterman L, Eipper B, Hubbard A. Dynamics of endogenous ATP7A (Menkes protein) in intestinal epithelial cells: copper-dependent redistribution between two intracellular sites. Am J Physiol Gastrointest Liver Physiol. 2007;292(4):G1181–94.
18. Coffey AJ, Durkie M, Hague S, et al. A genetic study of Wilson's disease in the United Kingdom. Brain. 2013;136(Pt 5):1476–87.
19. Wilson SA. Progressive lenticular degeneration: a familial nervous disease associated with cirrhosis of the liver. Brain. 1912;34:295–509.
20. Cumings J. The effects of B.A.L. in hepatolenticular degeneration. Brain. 1951;74:10–22.
21. Bull PC, Thomas GR, Rommens JM, Forbes JR, Cox DW. The Wilson disease gene is a putative copper transporting P-type ATPase similar to the Menkes gene. Nat Genet. 1993;5(4):327–37.
22. Tanzi RE, Petrukhin K, Chernov I, et al. The Wilson disease gene is a copper transporting ATPase with homology to the Menkes disease gene. Nat Genet. 1993;5(4):344–50.
23. Yamaguchi Y, Heiny ME, Gitlin JD. Isolation and characterization of a human liver cDNA as a candidate gene for Wilson disease. Biochem Biophys Res Commun. 1993;197(1):271–7.
24. Hellman NE, Kono S, Mancini GM, Hoogeboom AJ, De Jong GJ, Gitlin JD. Mechanisms of copper incorporation into human ceruloplasmin. J Biol Chem. 2002;277(48):46632–8.
25. Wilson Disease Mutation Database. http://www.medicalgenetics.med.ualberta.ca/wilson/index.php.
26. Usta J, Wehbeh A, Rida K, et al. Phenotype-genotype correlation in Wilson disease in a large Lebanese family: association of c.2299insC with hepatic and of p. Ala1003Thr with neurologic phenotype. PLoS One. 2014;9(11):e109727.
27. Wu ZY, Lin MT, Murong SX, Wang N. Molecular diagnosis and prophylactic therapy for presymptomatic Chinese patients with Wilson disease. Arch Neurol. 2003;60(5):737–41.
28. Yoshida K, Furihata K, Takeda S, et al. A mutation in the ceruloplasmin gene is associated with systemic hemosiderosis in humans. Nat Genet. 1995;9(3):267–72.

29. Roeser HP, Lee GR, Nacht S, Cartwright GE. The role of ceruloplasmin in iron metabolism. J Clin Invest. 1970;49(12):2408–17.
30. Gunther MR, Hanna PM, Mason RP, Cohen MS. Hydroxyl radical formation from cuprous ion and hydrogen peroxide: a spin-trapping study. Arch Biochem Biophys. 1995;316(1):515–22.
31. Mufti AR, Burstein E, Csomos RA, et al. XIAP is a copper binding protein deregulated in Wilson's disease and other copper toxicosis disorders. Mol Cell. 2006;21(6):775–85.
32. Gao B, Bataller R. Alcoholic liver disease: pathogenesis and new therapeutic targets. Gastroenterology. 2011;141(5):1572–85.
33. Min HK, Kapoor A, Fuchs M, et al. Increased hepatic synthesis and dysregulation of cholesterol metabolism is associated with the severity of nonalcoholic fatty liver disease. Cell Metab. 2012;15(5):665–74.
34. Paris I, Dagnino-Subiabre A, Marcelain K, et al. Copper neurotoxicity is dependent on dopamine-mediated copper uptake and one-electron reduction of aminochrome in a rat substantia nigra neuronal cell line. J Neurochem. 2001;77(2):519–29.
35. Tjaard Hoogenraad U. Wilson disease: major problems in neurology. Philadelphia: W .B. Saunders Company; 1996.

Chapter 2
Diagnosis Confirmation and Screening of Wilson Disease

Marinos Pericleous, Claire Kelly, and Michael L. Schilsky

Introduction

Wilson disease (WD) is a rare disorder of impaired copper metabolism whose underlying defect is in the hepatocytes in the liver. The inability to excrete normal quantities of copper in excess of metabolic needs eventually leads to copper overload with pathologic effects mainly in the liver and later in the central nervous system. The first report of WD and its associated neuro-hepatic presentation was described more than 100 years ago by

M. Pericleous · C. Kelly
Department of Gastroenterology and Hepatology, Royal Surrey County Hospital, Surrey, UK

Department of Clinical and Experimental Medicine, University of Surrey, Surrey, UK

M. L. Schilsky (✉)
Division of Digestive Diseases and Transplant and Immunology, Departments of Medicine and Surgery, Yale University, New Haven, CT, USA
e-mail: michael.schilsky@yale.edu

M. L. Schilsky (ed.), *Management of Wilson Disease*, Clinical Gastroenterology, https://doi.org/10.1007/978-3-319-91527-2_2

Kinnier Wilson as part of his MD thesis [1]. The disorder is inherited in an autosomal recessive Mendelian fashion [2, 3]. This implies that patients must inherit one abnormal allele on chromosome 13 from each parent. The prevalence of WD is estimated to be around 1:30,000 [4]. A defect on chromosome 13 in the *ATP7B* gene is responsible for WD. ATP7B is a copper-transporting protein primarily expressed in liver cells (hepatocytes) [5–11], and therefore defective function of this protein leads to excess copper accumulation in liver cells. For this reason, the first expression of WD is typically related to the liver, occurring in the first and second decades of life. Neurologic and psychiatric manifestations typically present later on, and other organs of the body may be affected as well. In this chapter, we will focus on in whom to consider a diagnosis of WD (Table 2.1), how we establish a diagnosis of WD, and discuss screening of other family members for this disorder once the diagnosis of WD is established.

Patients to Test for Wilson Disease

It is important to know when to consider the diagnosis and initiate the appropriate testing for WD. Given the inherited

Table 2.1 When to consider a diagnosis of Wilson disease

Unexplained abnormal liver function tests
Unexplained neurologic symptoms including tremor and other involuntary movements such us the ones seen in Parkinson's disease
Unexplained psychiatric presentations
Unexplained behavioral and personality changes
In children who underperform at school and there is no other explanation, e.g., neglect
In patients with incidental finding of Kayser-Fleischer rings on a routine eye exam
Unexplained hemolytic anemia
In family members of a patient with known or newly diagnosed Wilson disease

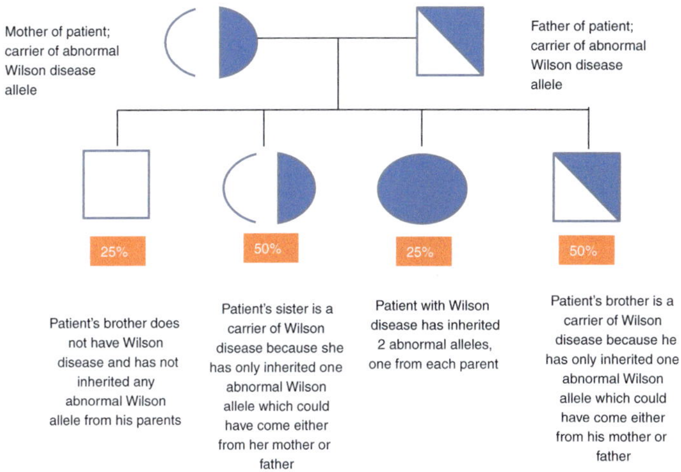

FIGURE. 2.1 Wilson disease is an autosomal recessive condition which means that a patient must inherit two abnormal alleles with *ATP7B* mutations from his/her parents. If both parents are carriers as shown in this pedigree, then there is a 25% chance that the offspring will have Wilson disease, 50% chance that the offspring will be a carrier like the parents, and a 25% chance that the offspring will not inherit any abnormal alleles in relation to Wilson disease. Male and female offspring are affected by this mode of inheritance at equal levels. It should be noted that in this pedigree, circles represent females, squares represent males, half-shaded shapes indicate that a person is a carrier, and a fully shaded shape indicate that a person is affected by Wilson disease

nature of this disorder as autosomal recessive, all siblings and primary relatives should be considered for testing (Fig. 2.1). In young children in whom the diagnosis is established, parents should be tested for WD as infrequently there are some families in which parent and child are affected. Other patients in whom WD should be considered are those with unexplained liver disease, with early onset of neurologic symptoms typical of Parkinson's disease, with neurologic findings such as tremor and who have abnormal liver tests, and with mood disorders and abnormal liver tests or neurologic findings. In addition, there are rare patients with unusual findings such as the fortuitous identification of Kayser-Fleischer rings on a routine eye exam or investigation of hemolytic anemia or aminoaciduria

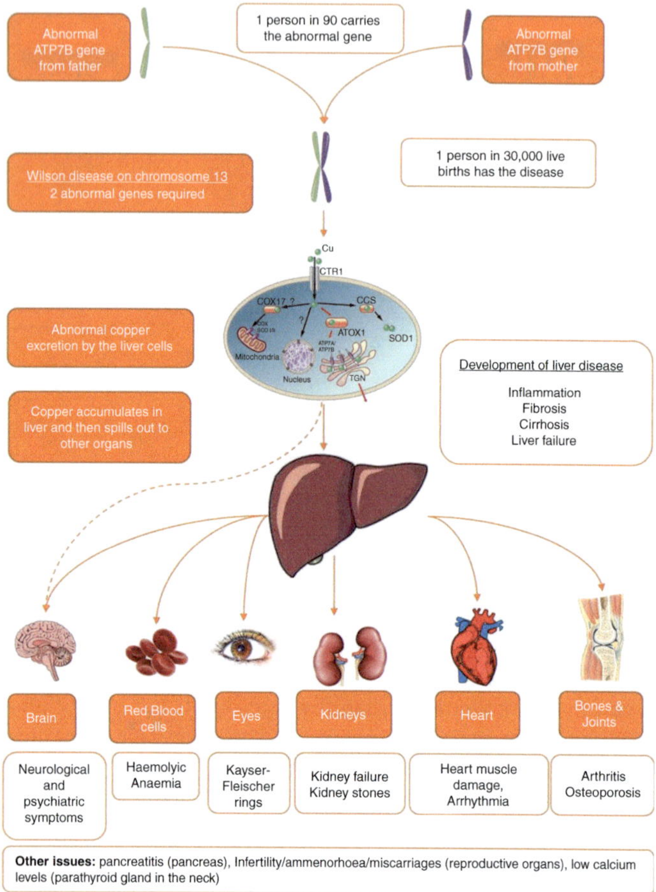

FIGURE. 2.2 Wilson disease is an autosomal recessive multisystem disease resulting from excess copper. Failure of the ATPase copper transporter in the liver, ATP7B, leads to excess amounts of copper in the liver and later in the circulation which is deposited in the peripheral tissues and central nervous system. A proportion of patients present primarily with neuropsychiatric symptoms without clinical findings of significant liver disease

(Fig. 2.2). Each of these categories is considered separately below in more detail, as well as the approach to testing needed to establish a diagnosis of WD.

Liver Disease and Extrahepatic Involvement in Wilson Disease

Unexplained liver disease is one of the more common reasons to seek a diagnosis of WD as liver disease is most often the earliest manifestation of WD. A separate chapter is devoted to the signs and symptoms of liver disease in WD and treatment for this, and therefore we will focus this section on the specific findings seen and diagnosis. As the liver is unable to excrete excess copper, this metal begins to accumulate and affects liver function. Abnormalities of the liver may range from abnormal liver tests to cirrhosis to overt liver failure. Liver tests commonly performed on biochemical analysis of blood include alanine aminotransferase (ALT), aspartate aminotransferase (AST), alkaline phosphatase (ALP), gamma-glutamyl transferase (GGT or "gamma-GT"), bilirubin, albumin, and clotting studies, i.e., prothrombin time (PT) or international normalized ratio (INR). Elevated levels of ALT and AST above the laboratories' normal range indicate a degree of inflammation (hepatitis) from damage to the liver cells (hepatocytes). The ALT is more specific to the liver than the AST since the latter is also found in the muscle. ALP is found in the bile ducts (the drainage system of bile within the liver), and its combination with GGT can indicate injury of bile ducts or physical blockage. A raised GGT can also potentially indicate toxic injury to the liver, as can occur with alcohol and following drug reactions. Bilirubin is a pigment created by the liver from recycled red blood cells, and it is found in abundance in bile. Jaundice occurs when accumulated bilirubin pigment alters skin coloration and can be caused by liver damage or blockage or injury of the bile ducts.

The liver is also responsible for synthesizing and exporting into the circulation of many proteins such as albumin and clotting factors. Albumin is an important molecule that functions as a carrier of other molecules and as a factor that maintains the body's fluid balance. A damaged liver will produce lower levels of albumin which can lead to swelling, especially in the lower limbs (peripheral edema), and fluid accumulation in the abdomen (ascites). Clotting factors are important proteins that ensure appropriate clot formation that is an important part of wound healing. A damaged liver will produce less of these factors which may lead to excessive bruising or predispose the patient to bleeding. The inability of a damaged liver to produce these useful proteins is called "impaired synthetic function," and measuring levels of the protein or indirectly the function of the protein to aid clotting (prothrombin time or the INR) helps to determine the degree of liver dysfunction.

In some circumstances WD may present in a way that it overlaps with other liver disorders. For instance, some pediatric patients have serum markers that overlap with autoimmune hepatitis and are treated for this disorder. In this setting, failure of liver tests to improve with treatment directed at the autoimmune hepatitis should prompt further consideration of WD. Another feature of WD that overlaps with other liver disorders is the accumulation of hepatic fat (steatosis) as one of the earliest findings of liver disease in WD, so the diagnosis should be considered in patients with nonalcoholic fatty liver disease or with steatohepatitis, fatty liver disease with inflammation. WD must also be considered in the setting of acute liver failure (ALF), and this is discussed separately below.

The Neuropsychiatric Manifestations of Wilson Disease: More than Meets the Eye

In his original publication, Kinnier Wilson coined the term "progressive lenticular degeneration" which described the degenerative changes observed at the lens-shaped lenticular nucleus (or lentiform nucleus) in the brain [1]. Anatomically, the lenticular nucleus is composed of the putamen and the globus pallidus which are areas within the basal ganglia of the brain. The role of the lenticular nucleus is to orchestrate body movements which have been initiated by other parts of the brain. This ensures that any motor activity of the body is smoothly coordinated. WD leads to the accumulation of excess copper in the basal ganglia and other areas of the brain such as the midbrain, pons, thalami, and cerebelli. Though other areas of the brain have copper, the basal ganglia appear more susceptible to injury. This explains the movement and speech disorders often observed in WD patients [12]. It is believed that 40% of patients with WD will present with neurological signs [13]. The progressive inability to control movement may lead to long-term disability and inability to cope with activities of daily living. Patients who present with neuropsychiatric symptoms are usually older, and a majority already have advanced liver disease, including cirrhosis [14].

Tremor

The tremor of WD is usually present in the hands and arms, but many parts of the body may be affected. The tremor is usually proximal, low frequency, and high amplitude and has been described as coarse and sometimes has a wing-beating appearance [15]. The tremor can be intermittent, present symmetrically on both sides of the body, or unilateral. The tremor may be unresponsive to dopaminergic medication (such as those used for Parkinson's disease) or alcohol, which often dampens essential tremor [16]. If tremor is present and there is any evidence of liver disease on exam or on biochemical testing, then a diagnosis of WD must be considered.

The Cranial Nerves

The cranial nerves are responsible for smelling, eyesight and eye movements, tasting, saliva production, facial movement and sensation, balance, hearing, talking, swallowing, and head and tongue movement. In WD, several of these 12 cranial nerves can be affected in clusters, or there may be involvement of one in isolation [16, 17]. Cranial nerve involvement can explain why some patients may present with involuntary blinking, abnormal neck posture, facial grimacing, speech difficulties, drooling, and difficult swallowing. This involuntary and uncoordinated change in muscle tone – often painful – is called dystonia and may be commonly encountered in patients with WD with neurologic symptoms. There are several types of dystonia, and these are summarized in Table 2.1. In patients with cranial nerve findings or with dystonia and abnormal liver tests, then WD must be considered.

The Cerebellum

The part of the brain known as the cerebellum plays an important role in coordinating voluntary motor activity such as walking and speech, and it is also involved in balance and posture control. The cerebellum is involved in cognition and affect, so patients with cerebellar injury may present with anxiety, depression, and impaired language skills [18, 19]. WD is known to affect the cerebellum, and the resulting symptoms that may be found are outlined in Table 2.2.

Psychiatric Symptoms

Up to 30–40% patients with WD will present with behavioral or psychiatric symptoms, and 20% would have seen a psychiatrist prior to the diagnosis [4, 20]. Most commonly, patients will present with affective disorders involving their mood such as depression, mania, and bipolar disorder as well as behavioral disorders which can include anxiety, obsessive-compulsive disorder (OCD), and attention deficit hyperactivity disorder (ADHD) [20]. Delayed diagnosis is not unusual, especially when symptoms are subtle and patients may be

TABLE 2.2 List of neurologic diagnoses frequently seen in patients with Wilson disease

Collective term	Neurologic diagnosis	Clinical sign/presentation
Dystonia	Blepharospasm	Involuntary blinking and twitching of eyelids
	Torticollis: painful spasm of neck muscles	Abnormal posture of the neck
	Limb and fascial muscle dystonia	Contractures and twisting of limb muscles, grimacing, abnormal jaw posture
	Voice dystonia	Strained and effortful speech, hoarse voice, loss of voice (aphonia)
	Oropharyngeal dystonia including lingual dystonia	Drooling, dysphagia
	Dystonic tremor	Irregular oscillation of any part of the body
	Status dystonicus or dystonic storm	Severe muscle spasms anywhere in the body which can involve any muscle including those of swallowing and breathing
Dysarthria (difficulty speaking)	Cerebellar dysarthria	Scanning, staccato speech
	Pseudobulbar/extrapyramidal dysarthria	Slurred speech
	Bulbar dysarthria	Nasal/slurred speech

TABLE 2.2 (continued)

Collective term	Neurologic diagnosis	Clinical sign/presentation
Cerebellar disorders	Dysdiadochokinesis	Unable to perform rapid, sequential movements
	Ataxia	Impaired movement coordination (limb and truncal)
	Nystagmus	Rapid and involuntary eye movements
	Intention tremor	Trembling when a voluntary movement is attempted
	Staccato speech	As above
	Hypotonia	Reduced muscle tone leading to "floppy" appearance
Basal ganglia dysfunction	Chorea	Involuntary dance-like movements
	Athetosis	Involuntary writhing movements
Peripheral neuropathy	Small fiber peripheral neuropathy (including autonomic neuropathy, dysautonomia)	Numbness, pins and needles, impaired balance, impaired control of blood pressure, gastrointestinal problems, bladder problems, dizziness
Other	Seizures (focal or generalized)	Convulsions
	Micrographia	Small handwriting

misdiagnosed at a young age as poor school performers or with puberty-related behavior abnormalities. Older patients may be misdiagnosed with Parkinsonism or dementia. Table 2.3 summarizes the spectrum of psychiatric manifestations encountered in patients with WD. If any of these are present in concert with liver disease, then WD must be excluded.

Other Organs Involved in Wilson Disease

Damage due to copper in WD is not limited to the liver, and other organs of the body, in particular in the brain, may be affected (discussed in the next section). Aside from the brain, there may be involvement of other organs due to excess copper. These include the eyes, kidneys, heart, gonads, gallbladder, joints/bones, heart, and red blood cells (Fig. 2.2 and Table 2.4) [4, 21–32].

TABLE 2.3 List of psychiatric diagnoses often seen in patients with Wilson disease

Psychiatric/behavioral manifestations of Wilson disease	
Falling behind with school	Hallucinations
Personality and behavioral change	Deliberate self-harm
Depression/mania/bipolar disorder	Euphoria
Anxiety	Apathy
Mood changes	Suicidal ideation
Memory impairment	Hypersexuality
Paranoia	Disinhibition
Schizophrenia/psychosis	Catatonia
Delusions	Obsessive-compulsive disorder

Table 2.4 Nonhepatic nonnervous system manifestations of Wilson disease

Joints/bones	Premature arthritis Arthralgia Chondrocalcinosis
Pancreas	Pancreatitis
Pituitary	Gigantism Infertility Impotence
Heart	Cardiomyopathy Arrhythmias
Gonads	Impotence Infertility Abortions
Kidneys	Renal stones Renal tubular acidosis
Bone marrow and red blood cells	Hemolytic anemia

Confirming the Diagnosis

As discussed above, WD may present with a wide range of clinical presentations and present clinically in younger or even older patients. The diagnosis can be challenging at times even for the most observant physician, but cannot be made unless considered. For this reason, a formal scoring system was created to help physicians determine if their evaluation has established a diagnosis of WD or if further testing is still needed. This scoring system, known as the Leipzig score, was developed at a meeting of experts on WD held in Leipzig, Germany [33]. The Leipzig score utilizes a combination of clinical and biochemical parameters, each with a weighted score for the elements of the testing. It was also the first scoring system to include molecular genetic testing for *ATP7B* mutations as one of the elements of the testing.

In setting out to evaluate a patient using the Leipzig score, a reasonable diagnostic approach should begin with noninvasive parameters such as serological and urine tests as well as slit-lamp examination. If necessary, these could be followed by a liver biopsy for histological evaluation and genetic analysis. The exception for doing the molecular testing as a first order test is when using this for screening of siblings for WD when the mutations have been identified in a patient (see below). An algorithmic approach to this testing is outlined in the guidelines published by the American Association for the Study of Liver Disease [30]. Some of the individual components of the Leipzig score used for WD testing are discussed separately below.

Slit-Lamp Examination for Kayser-Fleischer (KF) Rings

The German physicians Bernhard Kayser and Bruno Fleischer first described corneal deposits in the eye (Kayser-Fleischer rings) in 1902 and 1903, but it was not until years later, in 1922, that these deposits in Descemet's membrane of the cornea were composed of copper (Fig. 2.3) [34, 35]. Approximately 95% of patients who primarily present with neurological and/or psychiatric WD will have KF rings, whereas KF rings will be absent in approximately 50% of

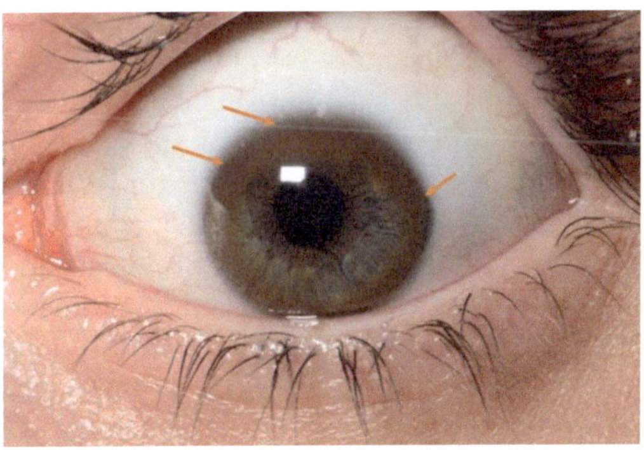

FIGURE. 2.3 Kayser-Fleischer ring in a 25-year-old with Wilson disease

patients presenting with liver disease [36, 37]. KF rings may also be absent in younger patients, and testing for these is not typically needed before the age of 5 years. In some cases, KF rings may be seen by the naked eye on a bedside examination; nevertheless, a slit examination by an experienced ophthalmologist is always required to confirm their presence as other findings such as arcus may be confused for KF rings. There are rare instances where KF rings can be found in other liver disorders where bile flow is obstructed, such as primary biliary cholangitis and primary sclerosing cholangitis [38, 39]. Because of these rare happenings and because there may be false-positive reports of KF rings, the finding of KF rings should not be used in isolation to make the diagnosis of WD.

A slit-lamp examination can also identify the presence of another less common finding of sunflower cataracts, which are also caused by copper deposition in the center of the lens of the eye. This finding also supports the diagnosis of WD [40].

Serum Ceruloplasmin

Ceruloplasmin (from Latin caeruleus = dark blue and Greek πλάσμα-plasma = formation) is the main copper-carrying protein in the human blood. It is also an acute-phase reactive protein which means that it can be elevated when there is inflammation in the body. Ceruloplasmin is sensitive to estrogen, and its levels may increase during pregnancy or in patients who are taking supplementary hormonal therapy with estrogens. Ceruloplasmin also has antioxidant properties [41], but more importantly, it plays a role in iron metabolism where it serves as a ferroxidase. When the peptide for ceruloplasmin is initially produced in liver cells, it is without copper and is also known as "apo"ceruloplasmin. When ceruloplasmin contains bound copper, it is known as "holo"ceruloplasmin (six copper atoms per molecule). The association of a low ceruloplasmin in the circulation of patients with WD was made in 1952 by Scheinberg and Gitlin [42]. Low ceruloplasmin levels in ~20% of asymptomatic carriers, heterozygote individuals without WD, were also reported for the first time in 1968 [43].

Approximately, 85–90% of homozygous patients with WD will have low ceruloplasmin levels (<0.2 g/L OR 20 mg/dL or 200 mg/L, depending on the range of normal for the individual laboratory) [44–46]. Extremely low levels (<0.05 g/L or < 5 mg/dL or < 50 mg/L) are more strongly associated with the diagnosis of WD. The mechanism for having low ceruloplasmin levels in WD is related to the ineffective placement of copper into apoceruloplasmin and the shorter half-life of apoceruloplasmin in the circulation due to more rapid degradation of this form of the protein compared to holoceruloplasmin. Ceruloplasmin levels may also be low in patients with very poor liver function where all proteins produced by the liver are low, when there is severe protein loss from the kidney or the gut and in states of copper deficiency. The causes of a low serum ceruloplasmin level are shown in Table 2.6.

There are some patients with WD who have normal ceruloplasmin levels [36, 37, 47–50]. Therefore ceruloplasmin cannot be used in isolation for establishing or excluding the diagnosis of WD.

Free (Unbound) Serum Copper

Free copper levels are often measured by the labs as part of the diagnostic workup of patients with suspected WD; however, its measurement is particularly useful in the clinical setting as marker of treatment monitoring, providing the clinician with an insight into the effectiveness of de-coppering therapy and compliance with prescribed treatment. Most commercial assays measure total serum or plasma copper that includes both copper bound to apoceruloplasmin (to form holoceruloplasmin) and unbound circulating copper, or non-ceruloplasmin copper. It is only the unbound copper that is actively involved in copper metabolism as this is the copper that is used by cells as cofactors in metabolism and can deposit in the liver and in organs outside the liver when present in excess. As most conventional assays do not provide a direct measurement of unbound copper, its concentrations can be measured indirectly using:

$$\text{Free}(\text{Unbound})\text{Serum Copper} = \\ [\text{Serum Copper in } \mu g / \text{L}] - [3.15 \times \text{Serum Ceruloplasmin in mg} / \text{dL}]$$

Normally, levels are less than 25 μg/dL, and in patients who are overtreated that may become copper-depleted, levels are less than 5 μg/dL. Serum levels of unbound copper are not part of the Leipzig score since there are difficulties in many patients with this estimate using commercial assays. This is discussed further in the chapter on treatment monitoring.

Twenty-Four-Hour Urinary Copper

Unlike unbound serum copper, 24-h urinary copper levels are one of the elements of the Leipzig score. Twenty-four-hour urinary copper excretion of >100 μg/24 h (>1.6 μmol/24 h) is strongly suggestive of the diagnosis in symptomatic patients, but approximately a quarter of confirmed asymptomatic cases of WD will have lower or normal levels [48, 51, 52]. It is generally accepted that levels >40 μg or > 0.6 μmol (or > 600 nmol) should raise suspicion of WD and lead to further investigations. Special cases include patients with chronic liver disease who may have higher levels but typically not >100 μg/24 h and heterozygotes for WD who may have intermediately elevated levels of 24-h urinary copper. Patients with proteinuria and acute liver failure may present with falsely elevated levels of urine copper. The collection of urine requires a metal-free container and should be a full 24-hour collection.

Genetic Analysis: Testing for ATP7B Mutations

Molecular testing is a useful adjunct in establishing the diagnosis of WD in patients with unexplained liver disease but also the first-line investigation for screening the siblings of a patient with a secure diagnosis of WD [30]. Patients with WD inherit two defective *ATP7B* alleles (one from each parent). The inherited gene may be mutated at the same location (homozygous) or at different location on *ATP7B* (compound heterozygote). Most patients are compound heterozygotes. To date, there are several mutations identified often with a geographical predilection [53]. It is possible that some mutations may be more pathogenic than others, with large deletions or changes that produce absence of functional ATP7B protein, though good data on genotype and phenotype correlation is not definitive. There may be some mutations with partial function where disease is speculated to be milder or later in its onset. Interestingly, patients with the same mutations may present differently (phenotype). We believe this is due to differences in their dietary intake of copper as well as other modifying factors, such as resistance to oxidative injury or different regenerative capacity of their livers.

Genetic analysis may involve genotyping of the whole *ATP7B* gene and looking for more than 600 areas of potential abnormalities or even exploring for new mutations not previously described. Whereas previously, the process of whole-gene sequencing was lengthy and technically challenging, recent technologic advancements have allowed for quicker, elaborate, and more affordable analysis. As certain mutations were shown to be more prevalent in particular geographical areas and specific populations, allele-specific probes can be used to look for predominant mutations. Identification of one mutation will support the diagnosis of WD, and two mutations will establish it. This is reflected in the Leipzig scoring system with different point designations for these findings (see Table 2.5).

Liver Biopsy: Histology and Hepatic Copper Concentration

When noninvasive tests are still not conclusive or when staging of liver disease is required, then a liver biopsy should be requested. The biopsy can provide information about the extent of histological damage including the degree of scarring (fibrosis) or the presence of cirrhosis (end-stage liver scarring). Histological findings in WD may resemble those seen in fatty liver disease, nonalcoholic steatohepatitis, and autoimmune hepatitis. Moreover, a liver biopsy can be used for copper staining and for

TABLE 2.5 The Leipzig scoring system for Wilson disease consists of seven parameters, and a score of ≥4 can establish the diagnosis

(1) Kayser-Fleischer rings	
Present	2
Absent	0
(2) Neurologic symptoms or typical imaging at brain magnetic resonance imaging	
Severe	2
Mild	1
Absent	0
(3) Serum ceruloplasmin	
Normal (>0.2 g/L)	0
0.1–0.2 g/L	1
<0.1 g/L	2
(4) Coombs negative hemolytic anemia	
Present	1
Absent	0
(5) Liver copper (in the absence of cholestasis)	
>x5 ULN (>4 μmol/g)	2
0.8–4 μmol/g	1
Normal (<0.8 μmol/g)	−1
Rhodanine-positive granules (if no quantifiable copper available)	1
(6) Urinary copper (in the absence of acute hepatitis)	
Normal	0
1–2x ULN	1
>2 ULN	2
Normal but >5x ULN after D-penicillamine	2
(7) Mutation analysis	
On both chromosomes	4
On one chromosome	1
No mutation detected	0
Total score:	
4 or more = diagnosis established	
3 = diagnosis possible, more tests needed	
2 or less = diagnosis very unlikely	

From Ferenci et al. [33]

Patients with a score of <4 should complete the appropriate testing to exclude the diagnosis

Table 2.6 Conditions which may lead to low serum ceruloplasmin levels

Wilson disease
Heterozygote carriers of the *APT7B* gene (Wilson disease)
Menkes disease (ATP7A defect)
Malnourishment leading to copper deficiency
Malabsorption, e.g., gastric bypass surgery
Protein-losing enteropathy/nephropathy
Aceruloplasminemia
Excessive zinc administration
Impaired synthetic liver function; end-stage liver disease

quantifying the content of dry copper in the liver. This is in fact one of the parameters of the Leipzig score (Table 2.5).

Normally the dry copper concentration in the liver does not exceed 50 μg (0.8 μmol)/g dry weight. Heterozygous patients will often have levels 50–250 μg (0.8–4 μmol)/g dry weight and homozygous patients often >250 μg (4 μmol)/g dry weight [54]. It has been reported that the sensitivity and specificity using a cutoff of >250 μg (4 μmol)/g dry weight of the diagnosis of WD are 83% and 99%, respectively [55]. Just like the other diagnostic tests for WD, interpretation of results should be taken in the context of the biochemical findings, medical history, and clinical presentation. It should be noted that cholestatic conditions such as PBC and PSC may display higher-than-normal levels of dry weight liver copper, but these have specific histological findings that help establish the correct diagnosis.

Hemolysis (Breakdown of Red Blood Cells)

Patients with WD may present with hemolysis, a condition describing the breakdown of red blood cells (RBCs). This often leads to anemia and increased levels of bilirubin and the appearance of jaundice. Even though in many other chronic diseases hemolysis is driven by an autoimmune process (misdirected immune process), this does not appear to be the case in WD. Even though the exact mechanism is not fully understood, the hemolysis is probably due to toxic accumulation of copper in RBCs and the destabilizing effect of excess copper on the cell membranes. In some reported cases, hemolysis might be the first presenting feature in WD [4, 25–29]. The suggested workup for a patient with suspected hemolysis is shown in Table 2.7.

Imaging Tests

Several types of scans can be useful in identifying direct and indirect signs of chronic liver disease, including WD. Imaging investigations (scans) normally start by performing an ultrasound scan (USS) which is an excellent modality in identifying (a) changes in the outline of the liver (which could be

TABLE 2.7 Suggested workup for patients with suspected hemolysis

Parameter	**Findings/interpretation/rationale**
Coombs (or direct antiglobulin) test	Positive in autoimmune hemolysis, negative in Wilson disease
Reticulocyte count	Increased
Full blood count	Anemia
Iron studies	To identify cause of anemia
Vitamin B12	To identify cause of anemia
Folate levels	To identify cause of anemia
Thyroid function tests	To identify cause of anemia
Haptoglobin levels	Decreased
Unconjugated (indirect) bilirubin	Increased
Blood film/smear	May show fragments of red blood cells

suggestive of cirrhosis), (b) liver masses, (c) liver fat (steatosis), and (d) abnormal flow of blood in the main blood vessels within the liver. Cross-sectional imaging including computed tomography (CT) and magnetic resonance imaging (MRI) provide a better definition of the liver anatomy and are often used as second-line imaging investigations. A special type of MRI (MRCP) is the test of choice when suspecting issues with the biliary drainage of the liver and pancreas. Cross-sectional imaging is particularly useful in identifying signs such as (a) engorged/collateral blood vessels (varices), (b) blocked arteries and veins (thrombosis), (c) enlarged spleen (splenomegaly), and (d) fluid collection in the abdomen (ascites) which could allude to liver cirrhosis, high-pressure blood circulation in the liver (portal hypertension), higher risk of bleeding from ruptured varices, and liver cancer.

Cross-sectional imaging can be a useful adjunct for the diagnosis of WD, but copper itself cannot be seen on any imaging modality. Patients with neuropsychiatric presentations may display T2 hyperintensity in the brain's white matter, basal ganglia, and brainstem on magnetic resonance imaging (MRI). One of the commonly reported radiological findings is the panda sign where T2-weighted MRI sequences demonstrate the face of a giant panda in the midbrain of patients with neuropsychiatric WD [56]. This sign was previously regarded as pathognomonic of WD, but we now know that it can be also found in other conditions such as Japanese encephalitis and sarcoidosis. MRI scans of patients with purely hepatic disease are often normal. MRI is generally preferred to computed tomography (CT).

Acute Liver Failure Secondary to Wilson Disease

WD can uncommonly present with acute liver failure (ALF) in patients who have not been previously aware of having any pre-existing liver disease. According to the ALF study group data, approximately 1.2% (29/2436) of cases of ALF in the USA are due to WD [57]. Patients will commonly present with Coombs negative hemolytic anemia, progression to kidney failure from the tubular damage caused by the copper, deranged blood clotting, modest elevation of serum aminotransferases (<2000 IU/L), normal or low alkaline phosphatase (ALP) (<40 IU/L), and female predilection [30]. The combination of hepatic failure with hemolysis leads to elevated total bilirubin levels. A bilirubin: ALP ratio of >2 IU/L is an indirect indicator of WD in the context of ALF [30, 58, 59]. Serum ceruloplasmin is usually low, but reduced ceruloplasmin levels in ALF are not exclusive to WD. Serum ceruloplasmin levels can be normal in 15% of patients presenting with ALF secondary to WD [60]. Hepatic and urinary copper levels are usually greatly elevated and can support the diagnosis; however, these results are not always rapidly available. Uric acid levels may also be low. Physical examination may reveal KF rings in approximately 50% of these patients [59]. A rare but useful finding of a blue discoloration of the nails (*lunulae ceruleae*) may suggest WD [61]. Table 2.8 provides a summary of the commonest presenting features of WD in the setting of ALF. Treatment for stabilizing patients includes albumin dialysis, continuous hemofiltration, plasmapheresis, and plasma exchange, but ultimately these patients require liver transplantation. The management of patients presenting with ALF secondary to WD is discussed in more detail in different chapter of this book.

Family Screening

It is recommended that first-degree relatives of patients with WD should be screened for the disease using molecular genetic testing (described above) [4, 30]. These include siblings and offspring of the proband (first patient identified in the family with WD). The risk of a sibling having the disease follows Mendelian inheritance and is 25%, while the risk of being a carrier is 50%. Mutation-specific or haplotype screening should be undertaken for all siblings based on the probands' identified mutations. This method is quicker and more cost-effective than whole-genome sequencing. If two mutations (see Leipzig score; Table 2.5) or identical haplotype

Table 2.8 Summary of the main biochemical and clinical features of Wilson disease presenting in the context of acute liver failure

Female patient
Coombs negative hemolytic anemia
Rapid progression to kidney failure
Low/normal alkaline phosphatase (usually <40 IU/L)
Modest elevation of aminotransferases (usually <2000 IU/L)
Elevated total bilirubin
Raised bilirubin: ALP ratio (>2 IU/L)
Coagulopathy
Low serum ceruloplasmin
Elevated urinary copper
Elevated hepatic copper
Low uric acid levels
Kayser-Fleischer rings
Lunulae ceruleae

(patterns of sequences around the gene) is found, then the diagnosis of WD is established, and treatment should be considered. If genetic analysis is indeterminate for the siblings or if molecular testing is not available, then the standard investigations described above should be employed. Similarly, the children of the proband should be considered for noninvasive tests initially when they are older than 2 years of age and asymptomatic or sooner if symptomatic. The risk of the offspring of a proband having WD is believed to be 0.5% [4].

Conclusion

The diagnosis of WD can be established using the Leipzig scoring system developed to provide a diagnostic framework for clinicians. This scoring system uses clinical, biochemical, and molecular testing and provides an evidence-based structure for the diagnosis of patients. Consideration of WD in the appropriate patients, its prompt diagnosis and identification of the disease, and early treatment are associated with better clinical outcomes. Family screening is recommended for first-degree relatives of patients and may detect the disease prior to the appearance of signs or symptoms.

References

1. Compston A. Progressive lenticular degeneration: a familial nervous disease associated with cirrhosis of the liver, by S. A. Kinnier Wilson, (From the National Hospital, and the Laboratory of the National Hospital, Queen Square, London) Brain 1912: 34; 295–509. Brain. 2009;132(Pt 8):1997–2001.
2. Bearn AG, Kunkel HG. Abnormalities of copper metabolism in Wilson's disease and their relationship to the aminoaciduria. J Clin Invest. 1954;33(3):400–9.
3. Hall HC. La dégénérescence hépato-lenticulaire : maladie de Wilson, pseudo-sclérose. Paris: Masson; 1921. xi. p. 361.
4. European Association for Study of L. EASL clinical practice guidelines: Wilson's disease. J Hepatol. 2012;56(3):671–85.
5. Frydman M, Bonne-Tamir B, Farrer LA, Conneally PM, Magazanik A, Ashbel S, et al. Assignment of the gene for Wilson disease to chromosome 13: linkage to the esterase D locus. Proc Natl Acad Sci U S A. 1985;82(6):1819–21.
6. Vulpe C, Levinson B, Whitney S, Packman S, Gitschier J. Isolation of a candidate gene for Menkes disease and evidence that it encodes a copper-transporting ATPase. Nat Genet. 1993;3(1):7–13.
7. Chelly J, Tumer Z, Tonnesen T, Petterson A, Ishikawa-Brush Y, Tommerup N, et al. Isolation of a candidate gene for Menkes disease that encodes a potential heavy metal binding protein. Nat Genet. 1993;3(1):14–9.
8. Bull PC, Thomas GR, Rommens JM, Forbes JR, Cox DW. The Wilson disease gene is a putative copper transporting P-type ATPase similar to the Menkes gene. Nat Genet. 1993;5(4):327–37.
9. Mercer JF, Livingston J, Hall B, Paynter JA, Begy C, Chandrasekharappa S, et al. Isolation of a partial candidate gene for Menkes disease by positional cloning. Nat Genet. 1993;3(1):20–5.

10. Petrukhin K, Fischer SG, Pirastu M, Tanzi RE, Chernov I, Devoto M, et al. Mapping, cloning and genetic characterization of the region containing the Wilson disease gene. Nat Genet. 1993;5(4):338–43.
11. Tanzi RE, Petrukhin K, Chernov I, Pellequer JL, Wasco W, Ross B, et al. The Wilson disease gene is a copper transporting ATPase with homology to the Menkes disease gene. Nat Genet. 1993;5(4):344–50.
12. Glazebrook A. Wilson's disease. Edinburgh MJ. 1945;52(Feb.):83–7.
13. Stanbury JB, Wyngaarden JB, Fredrickson DS. The metabolic basis of inherited disease. 4th ed. New York/London: McGraw-Hill; 1978.
14. Schilsky ML, Tavill AS. Wilson disease. In: Schiff ER, Maddrey WC, Sorrell MF, editors. Schiff's diseases of the liver. 11th ed: Wiley-Blackwell; 2011.
15. Mahajan R, Zachariah U. Images in clinical medicine. Wing-beating tremor. N Engl J Med. 2014;371(1):e1.
16. LeWitt PA, Wilson's Disease CA. International neurology: Wiley-Blackwell; 2010. p. 644–7.
17. Choudhary N, Joshi L, Duggal A, Puri V, Khwaja GA. Isolated lingual involvement in Wilson's disease. J Neurosci Rural Pract. 2015;6(3):431–3.
18. De Smet HJ, Paquier P, Verhoeven J, Marien P. The cerebellum: its role in language and related cognitive and affective functions. Brain Lang. 2013;127(3):334–42.
19. Wolf U, Rapoport MJ, Schweizer TA. Evaluating the affective component of the cerebellar cognitive affective syndrome. J Neuropsychiatry Clin Neurosci. 2009;21(3):245–53.
20. Zimbrean PC, Schilsky ML. Psychiatric aspects of Wilson disease: a review. Gen Hosp Psychiatry. 2014;36(1):53–62.
21. Wang H, Zhou Z, Hu J, Han Y, Wang X, Cheng N, et al. Renal impairment in different phenotypes of Wilson disease. Neurol Sci. 2015;36(11):2111–5.
22. Weiss KH, Van de Moortele M, Gotthardt DN, Pfeiffenberger J, Seessle J, Ullrich E, et al. Bone demineralisation in a large cohort of Wilson disease patients. J Inherit Metab Dis. 2015;38(5):949–56.
23. Zhou XX, Qin HL, Li XH, Huang HW, Liang YY, Liang XL, et al. Characterizing brain mineral deposition in patients with Wilson disease using susceptibility-weighted imaging. Neurol India. 2014;62(4):362–6.
24. Rosenfield N, Grand RJ, Watkins JB, Ballantine TV, Levey RH. Cholelithiasis and Wilson disease. J Pediatr. 1978;92(2):210–3.

25. El Raziky MS, Ali A, El Shahawy A, Hamdy MM. Acute hemolytic anemia as an initial presentation of Wilson disease in children. J Pediatr Hematol Oncol. 2014;36(3):173–8.
26. Misztal S, Weiss B, Janukowicz-Lorenz H. Latent hemolytic syndrome in a case of Wilson' disease. Neurol Neurochir Pol. 1974;8(1):123–6.
27. Furrer HU, Tonz O. Acute hemolysis in morbus Wilson (author's transl). Z Kinderheilkd. 1974;118(2):147–62.
28. Buchanan GR. Acute hemolytic anemia as a presenting manifestation of Wilson disease. J Pediatr. 1975;86(2):245–7.
29. Forman SJ, Kumar KS, Redeker AG, Hochstein P. Hemolytic anemia in Wilson disease: clinical findings and biochemical mechanisms. Am J Hematol. 1980;9(3):269–75.
30. Roberts EA, Schilsky ML. American Association for Study of liver D. Diagnosis and treatment of Wilson disease: an update. Hepatology. 2008;47(6):2089–111.
31. Factor SM, Cho S, Sternlieb I, Scheinberg IH, Goldfischer S. The cardiomyopathy of Wilson's disease. Myocardial alterations in nine cases. Virchows Arch A Pathol Anat Histol. 1982;397(3):301–11.
32. Sinha S, Taly AB, Prashanth LK, Arunodaya GR, Swamy HS. Successful pregnancies and abortions in symptomatic and asymptomatic Wilson's disease. J Neurol Sci. 2004;217(1):37–40.
33. Ferenci P, Caca K, Loudianos G, Mieli-Vergani G, Tanner S, Sternlieb I, et al. Diagnosis and phenotypic classification of Wilson disease. Liver Int. 2003;23(3):139–42.
34. Siermerling E, Oloff H. Pseudosclerose mit Cornealring und doppelseitiger Scheinkatarakt, die nur bei seitlicher Beleuchtung sichtbar und die nach der Verletzung durch Kupfersplitter entstehenden Katarakten ahnlich ist. Klin Wochenschr. 1922;1:1087–9.
35. Jess A. Hornhautverkupferung in Form des Fleischerschen Pigmentringes bei der Pseudosklerose. Klin Mbl Augenheilk. 1922;69:218.
36. Gow PJ, Smallwood RA, Angus PW, Smith AL, Wall AJ, Sewell RB. Diagnosis of Wilson's disease: an experience over three decades. Gut. 2000;46(3):415–9.
37. Steindl P, Ferenci P, Dienes HP, Grimm G, Pabinger I, Madl C, et al. Wilson's disease in patients presenting with liver disease: a diagnostic challenge. Gastroenterology. 1997;113(1):212–8.
38. Fleming CR, Dickson ER, Hollenhorst RW, Goldstein NP, McCall JT, Baggenstoss AH. Pigmented corneal rings in a patient with primary biliary cirrhosis. Gastroenterology. 1975;69(1):220–5.

39. Mandal SK, Mandal L, Datta S, Bandyopadhyay D. Primary sclerosing cholangitis : an atypical presentation. J Assoc Physicians India. 2013;61(7):494–5.
40. Cairns JE, Williams HP, Walshe JM. "Sunflower cataract" in Wilson's disease. Br Med J. 1969;3(5662):95–6.
41. Atanasiu RL, Stea D, Mateescu MA, Vergely C, Dalloz F, Briot F, et al. Direct evidence of caeruloplasmin antioxidant properties. Mol Cell Biochem. 1998;189(1–2):127–35.
42. Scheinberg IH, Gitlin D. Deficiency of ceruloplasmin in patients with hepatolenticular degeneration (Wilson's disease). Science. 1952;116(3018):484–5.
43. Sternlieb I, Scheinberg IH. Prevention of Wilson's disease in asymptomatic patients. N Engl J Med. 1968;278(7):352–9.
44. Gibbs K, Walshe JM. A study of the caeruloplasmin concentrations found in 75 patients with Wilson's disease, their kinships and various control groups. Q J Med. 1979;48(191):447–63.
45. Brewer GJ, Yuzbasiyan-Gurkan V. Wilson disease. Medicine (Baltimore). 1992;71(3):139–64.
46. Stremmel W, Meyerrose KW, Niederau C, Hefter H, Kreuzpaintner G, Strohmeyer G. Wilson disease: clinical presentation, treatment, and survival. Ann Intern Med. 1991;115(9):720–6.
47. Cauza E, Maier-Dobersberger T, Polli C, Kaserer K, Kramer L, Ferenci P. Screening for Wilson's disease in patients with liver diseases by serum ceruloplasmin. J Hepatol. 1997;27(2):358–62.
48. Sanchez-Albisua I, Garde T, Hierro L, Camarena C, Frauca E, de la Vega A, et al. A high index of suspicion: the key to an early diagnosis of Wilson's disease in childhood. J Pediatr Gastroenterol Nutr. 1999;28(2):186–90.
49. Perman JA, Werlin SL, Grand RJ, Watkins JB. Laboratory measures of copper metabolism in the differentiation of chronic active hepatitis and Wilson disease in children. J Pediatr. 1979;94(4):564–8.
50. Martins da Costa C, Baldwin D, Portmann B, Lolin Y, Mowat AP, Mieli-Vergani G. Value of urinary copper excretion after penicillamine challenge in the diagnosis of Wilson's disease. Hepatology. 1992;15(4):609–15.
51. Giacchino R, Marazzi MG, Barabino A, Fasce L, Ciravegna B, Famularo L, et al. Syndromic variability of Wilson's disease in children. Clinical study of 44 cases. Ital J Gastroenterol Hepatol. 1997;29(2):155–61.
52. Gross JB Jr, Ludwig J, Wiesner RH, McCall JT, LaRusso NF. Abnormalities in tests of copper metabolism in primary sclerosing cholangitis. Gastroenterology. 1985;89(2):272–8.

53. Cocos R, Sendroiu A, Schipor S, Bohiltea LC, Sendroiu I, Raicu F. Genotype-phenotype correlations in a mountain population community with high prevalence of Wilson's disease: genetic and clinical homogeneity. PLoS One. 2014;9(6):e98520.
54. Scheinberg IH, Sternlieb I. Wilson's disease: W B Saunders; 1984.
55. Ferenci P, Steindl-Munda P, Vogel W, Jessner W, Gschwantler M, Stauber R, et al. Diagnostic value of quantitative hepatic copper determination in patients with Wilson's disease. Clin Gastroenterol Hepatol. 2005;3(8):811–8.
56. Jacobs DA, Markowitz CE, Liebeskind DS, Galetta SL. The "double panda sign" in Wilson's disease. Neurology. 2003;61(7):969.
57. Acute Liver Failure Study Group: Overview 2017 [Available from: http://www.utsouthwestern.edu/labs/acute-liver/overview/.
58. Korman JD, Volenberg I, Balko J, Webster J, Schiodt FV, Squires RH Jr, et al. Screening for Wilson disease in acute liver failure: a comparison of currently available diagnostic tests. Hepatology. 2008;48(4):1167–74.
59. Berman DH, Leventhal RI, Gavaler JS, Cadoff EM, Van Thiel DH. Clinical differentiation of fulminant Wilsonian hepatitis from other causes of hepatic failure. Gastroenterology. 1991;100(4):1129–34.
60. Schilsky ML. Diagnosis and treatment of Wilson's disease. Pediatr Transplant. 2002;6(1):15–9.
61. Kamate M, Prashanth GP, Gandhi S. A boy with sapphire thumbnails: Lunulae Ceruleae. Indian J Pediatr. 2014;81(7):737–8.

Chapter 3
Treatment Options for Wilson Disease

Claire Kelly, Marinos Pericleous, and Michael L. Schilsky

Treatment Options for Wilson Disease

Once a diagnosis of Wilson disease (WD) is established, treatment is needed. Treatment includes medical therapy directed at reducing the excess copper in the liver and other organs but also aimed at reducing symptoms of disease arising due to damage of the liver, brain, or other organs. Treatment also includes dietary management, physical or speech therapy if needed, or other interventions that try to enhance the quality of the patient's life. In those in

C. Kelly · M. Pericleous
Department of Gastroenterology and Hepatology, Royal Surrey County Hospital, Surrey, UK

Department of Clinical and Experimental Medicine, University of Surrey, Surrey, UK

M. L. Schilsky (✉)
Division of Digestive Diseases and Transplant and Immunology, Departments of Medicine and Surgery, Yale University, New Haven, CT, USA
e-mail: michael.schilsky@yale.edu

M. L. Schilsky (ed.), *Management of Wilson Disease*, Clinical Gastroenterology, https://doi.org/10.1007/978-3-319-91527-2_3

whom medical therapy is not possible due to liver failure or whom fail medical therapy, liver transplantation can be curative.

Treatment of patients diagnosed with WD can be divided into different stages and also has situations where there are special considerations:

1. *Initial therapy* that aims to remove excess copper from newly diagnosed symptomatic patients or *initial therapy* that aims to prevent signs and symptoms of disease in pre-symptomatic patients.
2. *Maintenance therapy* begins when stability of copper metabolism and symptomatic and continues lifelong.
3. Liver transplantation when medical therapy doesn't or will not work.
4. Other special circumstances: pregnancy and surgery (discussed in chapter 10).

Successful treatment of patients with WD requires a global view of the patient and the state of their disease, and for complex patients a multidisciplinary approach is often needed to achieve best outcomes. This chapter will focus mainly on drug therapy aimed at controlling the disordered copper metabolism which is the basis of this disorder but also on liver transplantation and when it is indicated. Treating other potential complications of WD, including those resulting from advanced liver disease, effects on the brain (neurologic and psychiatric disease), as well as dietary therapy to reduce intake and address nutritional needs that are important for overall health are addressed elsewhere in this book.

Drug therapy for WD was initially introduced in the 1950s, but the relatively rare nature of this condition and the manner in which the initial treatments were introduced (without dose-ranging studies, strict pharmacokinetic analysis, and head-to-head comparison studies between treatments to know which is best or safest) have left gaps in our knowledge of how best to use the currently available treatment regimens. Indeed, the choice of treatment for WD is often based on preferences of the treating physician or patient and may be guided by other factors (e.g., insurance coverage) as well as variable access to specific medications rather than by any available studies showing superiority of one treatment over another.

How then is a patient to choose between treatments? A working knowledge of the available medications and treatment options is the responsibility of the specialist who is prescribing the medications, but given the rarity of the disorder, it is likely that in any one community, there are not many treating physicians with experience. Patients and caregivers are therefore encouraged to learn more about their treatment options themselves and to seek further consultation at centers of excellence (designated by the patient-run Wilson disease Association, https://www.wilsonsdisease.org) where expert multidisciplinary teams are able to provide comprehensive consultation and make recommendations that incorporate the latest information, including participation in clinical trials.

A summary of the available oral therapies is shown in Table 3.1.

Drug Therapy

Dimercaprol (British Anti-Lewisite, BAL)

Dimercaprol (British anti-lewisite, BAL) was the first drug that successfully treated WD and provided dramatic improvement in patients with neurologic symptoms due to WD in whom no prior treatment was available. Recordings of some of the incredible responses to the treatments with this therapy are available [1]. BAL chelates (binds) and then causes

Table 3.1 Oral therapy for Adults with WD

Treatment	Dosing regimen	Mode of action
D-penicillamine	Usually 750–1000 mg in 3–4 divided doses	Chelator promoting urinary excretion of copper
Trientine	Usually 1000–1500 mg in 2–3 divided doses	Chelator promoting urinary excretion of copper
Zinc salts (gluconate, sulfate and acetate)	150 mg elemental zinc in three divided doses	Reduces copper absorption

removal of copper in the urine. This drug is rarely used now as it requires regular intramuscular injection and may cause a systemic hypersensitivity reaction and local sterile abscesses at the injection sites. The oral chelators D-penicillamine and trientine, discussed next, were developed in a bid to overcome the problems associated with BAL. A summary of the characteristics of these oral medications is shown in Table 3.2.

TABLE 3.2 Characteristics of comminly used therapies in adults for WD

Treatment	**Advantages**	**Disadvantages**
D-Penicillamine	Lengthy clinical experience Data supporting use Suitable for all presentations of WD	Frequency of side effects Hypersensitivity (fever and rash) Requires supplemental pyridoxine Marrow suppression Paradoxical neurological worsening during initiation of treatment Lupus-like syndrome Skin changes Colitis[a] Frequency of dosing
Trientine	Less side effects than D-penicillamine Suitable for all presentations of WD	Needs to be kept refrigerated Sideroblastic anemia Paradoxical neurological worsening during initiation of treatment Hemorrhagic gastritis[a] Duodenitis[a] Loss of taste Rash
Zinc salts	Well tolerated Neurological deterioration is uncommon	Gastrointestinal side effects Elevated lipase and/or amylase[a] Frequency of dosing Unclear if safe as monotherapy in hepatic disease

[a]Rare events

D-Penicillamine

D-Penicillamine was first used in WD in 1956 [2]. It acts by binding the copper and increasing its urinary excretion, but it may also induce metallothionein (a naturally occurring peptide that can safely bind copper) in the liver [3]. D-Penicillamine was shown to be useful in treating WD in many clinical studies [4–11]. In patients with liver disease, recovery of synthetic function of the liver and improvement in signs and symptoms related to WD can be seen in the initial 2–6 months of treatment, with even further recovery possible during the next year and beyond. There are even reports of advanced fibrosis (scarring in the liver) and cirrhosis improving on prolonged therapy [12]. In patients with neurologic WD, improvement of symptoms is often slower and may continue for a few years [6].

To improve tolerability, it is recommended to start with a low-dose regimen initially and slowly increase the dosage; starting with 125–250 mg/day that is increased by 250 mg every 4–7 days to a maximum of ~1500–2000 mg/day in 2–4 divided dosages in adults or to ~ 20 mg/kg in children. If taken with food, absorption of D-penicillamine is decreased [13], and therefore it is recommended to take this medication 1 h before or 2 h after meals. For children who cannot swallow capsules or for those with severe neurologic impairment and have difficulty swallowing and have either a gastric feeding tube or naso-enteral feeding tube, D-penicillamine is available in a liquid formulation. After successful treatment for a period of ~ 6–12 months during which time most excess circulating copper has been removed (see monitoring chapter for details of testing to follow while on treatment), the dose of D-penicillamine can be reduced by about 30–15% mg/kg for those who continue on D-penicillamine for maintenance therapy. Additionally, D-penicillamine interferes with vitamin B6 action; therefore supplemental pyridoxine should be provided (25–50 mg/day) as well to WD patients on D-penicillamine therapy.

While the majority of WD patients do well on treatment with d-penicillamine, unfortunately, worsening of neurologic symptoms may occur in some who are started on

D-penicillamine during their initial phase of treatment [6] or who restart this medication after long gaps in therapy. This neurological worsening is not unique to this drug and has been reported for other treatments used for WD, but it may be more frequent with D-penicillamine [14]. It is thought that worsening of neurologic symptoms or appearance of new neurologic symptoms following the initiation of WD treatment may be related to the mobilization of copper from sites within cells to the circulation given that the chelator-bound copper is still bioactive. However, it is important to remember that neurologic symptoms will certainly progress without treatment, and therefore the benefits of therapy outweigh risks. To reduce the risk of this occurring, many experts recommend a slow ramping up of the dose of D-penicillamine over a period of 1–2 months' time. Although some patients that do develop worsening of their neurologic status recover with continued use of D-penicillamine, it is recommended that the medication be stopped, or at least the dosage decreased when this occurs. There is a lack of clear evidence as to what is the best next step if neurological worsening occurs on treatment. One option is to consider changing treatment to include both zinc and a reduced dosage of chelating drug in combination (but given apart from each other, discussed below).

Another problem with D-penicillamine is the frequent occurrence of side effects, which leads to a change in treatment in around 25% of WD patients [7]. Side effects that are seen early on in treatment include hypersensitivity with fever and rash, marrow suppression, and, as noted above, early paradoxical neurological worsening. Other reactions include a lupus-like syndrome (rash, fever, kidney dysfunction), development of isolated kidney dysfunction with nephropathy (severe protein loss), a Wegener-like syndrome (inflammatory granulomas in the lung and other tissues), myasthenia gravis with muscular dysfunction, as well as dermatological changes including a keloid-like scar known as elastosis perforans serpiginosa and rarely colitis. In general, many of the side effects due to penicillamine are reversible when patients are changed to alternative therapies, trientine or zinc.

Copper-deficient states induced by high-dose D-penicillamine or prolonged treatment on standard dosages in those with strict restrictions of dietary copper. Overtreatment and a copper-deficient state can lead to iron overload in the liver and fatty change in liver cells, and this may contribute to liver injury independent of copper.

Trientine

Trientine is another copper chelator that was introduced in the late 1960s as an alternative to D-penicillamine for patients who could not use this drug. There is published evidence on the use of trientine, but clinical experience has outpaced this, with both suggesting trientine is as effective as D-penicillamine [7, 15–17]. Trientine seems to have fewer side effects and is useful in patients who are intolerant of D-penicillamine or where intolerance is more likely (history of renal disease, splenomegaly with severe thrombocytopenia, autoimmune tendencies) as well as for first-line therapy including in those with decompensated liver disease [18, 19].

The usual initial dose in adults is 20 mg/kg per day, rounded to the nearest 250 mg, given in two or three divided doses, with typical dosages of 900–2700 mg/day, with 900–1500 mg/day used for maintenance therapy in divided doses. The drug should be taken 1 h before or 2 h after meals. Trientine is not stable at high temperatures and should be refrigerated.

Trientine has few side effects. Neurological worsening with treatment initiation is seen with trientine but appears to be less common than with D-penicillamine [20]. No hypersensitivity reactions have been reported, but there is case reporting of a cutaneous drug reaction. Pancytopenia has rarely been reported. Lupus-like reactions have been reported, but almost all of these had previously had D-penicillamine. Rarely, trientine may cause hemorrhagic gastritis, colitis, duodenitis, loss of taste, and rash.

A reversible sideroblastic anemia has been described in case reports possibly because of the effects of trientine on iron metabolism [21, 22]. Trientine chelates iron, and this trientine-iron complex is nephrotoxic; thus iron supplementation should be avoided. Copper deficiency as a result of high-dose trientine over time can lead to iron overload in the liver, as is also seen with D-penicillamine [23].

Zinc

Zinc was found to be effective WD treatment in the early 1960s [24–27]. It works differently to the chelators described above. It interferes with the uptake of copper from the gastrointestinal tract through enterocyte metallothionein which binds copper, inhibiting its entry into the portal circulation [28, 29]. Once bound, the copper is lost as enterocytes are shed [6]. As copper also enters the gastrointestinal tract from saliva and gastric secretions, zinc treatment can generate a negative balance for copper and so remove stored copper [30].

Experience of zinc in the treatment of WD was gained through maintenance therapy after initial chelator use [31]. It has, however, been used as the initial treatment in patients who developed worsening neurologic symptoms with D-penicillamine, during pregnancy, in young children and in presymptomatic patients [5, 24, 25, 30–39]. The role of zinc in hepatic disease is controversial with conflicting reports over its efficacy. Deterioration has been reported, which proved fatal in one case [40, 41], but other reports suggest equivalent outcomes as is seen with D-penicillamine [42].

It has been suggested zinc may have a role as first-line therapy in patients with neurologic disease as there is no paradoxical worsening; however as it takes longer to reduce copper levels, the disease may progress on therapy. Thus, current guidelines recommend that all symptomatic patients diagnosed with WD should receive a chelating agent (D-penicillamine or trientine) [43, 44].

In presymptomatic patients, zinc is as effective as penicillamine but has less side effects [5].

Zinc is prescribed as zinc salts, with the common salts used being zinc sulfate, acetate, and gluconate. Zinc is dosed as milligrams of elemental zinc to allow consistent dosing across the different salts used though absorption of each may differ. The recommended dose in adults is 150 mg elemental zinc/day administered in three divided doses, 30 min before food. Taking zinc with food that contains phytates (a component of many grains in bread and cereals) interferes with absorption (a component of many grains in bread and cereals) [45]. Compliance with the three times per day dosage can be an issue, with twice daily still effective, but once daily is not [24]. Zinc has few side effects, with gastrointestinal issues the commonest which may be dependent on the salt employed with acetate and gluconate probably more tolerable than sulfate, but this varies with individuals. Elevations in serum lipase and/or amylase may occur, without clinical or radiologic evidence of pancreatitis. Neurological deterioration is uncommon with zinc [5, 46]. It is uncertain whether zinc is safe for patients with renal dysfunction.

Combination Therapy: Chelator and Zinc

The use of a combination of chelation therapy along with zinc (given separately) can be considered with the different mechanisms of action (preventing copper absorption and removal of excess copper, respectively) felt to have an advantage over either treatment alone.

Patients who present with decompensated cirrhosis have been treated with D-penicillamine [19, 47] or trientine [48], plus zinc. The chelator and zinc must be spread out throughout the day with usually 5–6 h between administrations of either drug, in order to avoid having the chelator bind the zinc. Typically zinc (50 mg elemental adult) is given as the first and third doses and trientine (500 mg) as the second and fourth doses. This is an intense treatment regimen in unwell patients which some will not respond to or tolerate [19, 47, 48]. Therefore, it is important these patients are treated in conjunction with a transplant center. Those who respond may be transitioned to full-dose zinc or full-dose trientine (or D-penicillamine) as monotherapy after 3–6 months. The combination of D-penicillamine and zinc may increase the risk for development of sideroblastic anemia.

Liver Transplantation

Liver transplantation may be the only option for patients who present with acute liver failure (occurs in ~5% with WD) and in those with decompensated liver disease who do not respond to medical therapy [49–54].

Patients with acute liver failure due to WD can have suggestive lab results including an aspartate aminotransferase (AST) to alanine aminotransferase (ALT) ratio >2.2, an alkaline phosphatase to bilirubin ratio <4, hemolytic anemia, and elevated serum copper >200 mcg/dL. These excess copper ions contribute to the hemolytic anemia.

Patients require treatment and stabilization in ICU and may well require urgent liver transplantation. Rapid removal of excess copper in the blood is crucial, and given the time for decoppering through drug therapy, various alternative methods have been used including hemodialysis, hemofiltration, albumin dialysis, plasma exchange, and molecular adsorbent recirculating system (MARS). A thorough workup for liver transplantation can occur in parallel with ICU care.

Transplantation corrects the hepatic metabolic defects of WD [55], and so patients do not require WD-specific treatment posttransplantation. While the posttransplantation outcomes for liver disease are excellent, transplantation is not recommended as a primary treatment for neurologic WD because any liver disease in these patients is stabilized by medical therapy, and outcomes with liver transplantation are not always beneficial [50, 54, 56–59]. Liver transplant assessment is covered in more detail in chapter 11.

Assessment of Therapy

An important assessment in the treatment of WD is 24-h urine copper excretion (see Table 3.3) which changes in pro-

TABLE 3.3 Typical results seen in monitoring of therapy in WD

	24-h urinary Cu	**NCC (calculated)**
Healthy individuals	20–50 μg/day	5–15 μg/dL
Untreated WD	100 μg/day (or greater)	Elevated (>25 μg/dL)
Penicillamine therapy (optimized)	200–500 μg/day	5–15 μg/dL
Trientine therapy (optimized)	200–500 μg/day	5–15 μg/dL
Zinc therapy (optimized)	<100 μg/day	5–15 μg/dL
Overtreated WD	<100 μg/day (chelators) <20 (zinc)	Very low
Poor compliance with therapy	<200 μg/day	Elevated (>25 μg/dL)

portion to the tissue stores depending on whether chelation or zinc therapy is used. Patients taking D-penicillamine or trientine should have 24-h urinary copper excretion values of 200–500 μg/day (3–8 mol/day); for patients on zinc, it should be <100 μg/day (1.2 mol/ day).

For patients on chelation therapy, elevated values for urine copper may suggest nonadherence to treatment. This is particularly important as lack of compliance with treatment leads to significant progression of liver disease and potentially liver failure within 1–12 months following discontinuation of treatment.

Adjunctive Therapy

Some authorities consider the use of other compounds in the treatment of WD. They can be used in conjunction with the therapies outlined above. They are not recommended in US or European guidelines due to a lack of clinical trial data supporting their use.

Curcumin

Curcumin is a naturally occurring compound in the spice turmeric. It could be helpful in WD through its antioxidant properties and may also have a role in copper chelation [60]. There is also experimental work looking at whether curcumin could have capacity to help increase the levels of protein expressed by the ATP7B gene and therefore improve copper export from cells [61]. There is not yet any data to support the clinical use of this compound, but some clinicians add it in to therapy after an individualized assessment.

Vitamin E

Vitamin E is an antioxidant. It has been found to be low in the blood and liver in patients with WD [62]. There have been reports of individuals improving symptomatically with supplementation, but there have also been reports of no correlation with low vitamin E and symptomatology. Therefore, its role is yet to be elucidated in the treatment of WD.

Chinese Herbal Medications

Various Chinese herbal medications (CHM) have been used in the management of WD, both alone and in conjunction with the therapies described earlier. A systematic review of nine randomized trials of varying quality of these medications found the evidence was not sufficient to make a clinical recommendation on their use [63].

Unmet Needs in Treatment of WD

There may be the opportunity to participate in clinical trials in discussion with a WD specialist due to unmet needs in the treatment of this condition.

Treatment can still take time (years) to improve symptoms and this can be compounded by worsening of neurologic symptoms seen in early treatment with existing chelators. A new formulation of tetrathiomolybdate (TTM) (bis-choline) which acts as first-in-class copper-protein-binding molecule is being investigated, with phase 2 data and extension phase reported [64, 65]. This compound was well tolerated and seems to be promising in addressing the paradoxical worsening of neurologic symptoms seen with other chelators. Phase 3 work is now underway (NCT03403205).

Patients can experience side effects on therapy which can impact on compliance, along with the multiple-dosing regimen of the currently available drugs. Clinical trials are ongoing to try to address these issues. The novel compound TTM described above also confers the advantage of once daily administration. Similarly, there are also trials in once daily administration of trientine [66].

There are issues regarding the affordability of existing therapy. This has led to attempts to develop biosimilar drugs. These are highly similar medicines to others already approved and have the same pharmaceutical quality, safety, and efficacy. Currently there is a clinical trial involving a biosimilar for trientine (EudraCT Number: 2016–003876-29).

References

1. Vilensky JA, Robertson WM, Gilman S. Denny-Brown, Wilson's disease, and BAL (British antilewisite [2,3-dimercaptopropanol]). Neurology. 2002;59(6):914–6.
2. Walshe JM. Wilson's disease; new oral therapy. Lancet. 1956 ;270:25–6.
3. Scheinberg IH, et al. Penicillamine may detoxify copper in Wilson's disease. Lancet. 1987;2(8550):95.
4. Walshe JM. Copper chelation in patients with Wilson's disease. A comparison of penicillamine and triethylene tetramine dihydrochloride. Q J Med. 1973;42(167):441–52.
5. Czlonkowska A, Gajda J, Rodo M. Effects of long-term treatment in Wilson's disease with D-penicillamine and zinc sulphate. J Neurol. 1996;243(3):269–73.
6. Brewer GJ, et al. Worsening of neurologic syndrome in patients with Wilson's disease with initial penicillamine therapy. Arch Neurol. 1987;44(5):490–3.
7. Weiss KH, et al. Efficacy and safety of oral chelators in treatment of patients with Wilson disease. Clin Gastroenterol Hepatol. 2013;11(8):1028–35 e1-2.

8. Sternlieb I. Copper and the liver. Gastroenterology. 1980;78(6):1615–28.
9. Grand RJ, Vawter GF. Juvenile Wilson disease: histologic and functional studies during penicillamine therapy. J Pediatr. 1975;87(6 Pt 2):1161–70.
10. Sass-Kortsak A. Wilson's disease. A treatable liver disease in children. Pediatr Clin N Am. 1975;22(4):963–84.
11. Falkmer S, Samuelson G, Sjolin S. Penicillamine-induced normalization of clinical signs, and liver morphology and histochemistry in a case of Wilson's disease. Pediatrics. 1970;45(2):260–8.
12. Bonis PA, Friedman SL, Kaplan MM. Is liver fibrosis reversible? N Engl J Med. 2001;344(6):452–4.
13. Schuna A, et al. Influence of food on the bioavailability of penicillamine. J Rheumatol. 1983;10(1):95–7.
14. Merle U, et al. Clinical presentation, diagnosis and long-term outcome of Wilson's disease: a cohort study. Gut. 2007;56(1):115–20.
15. Scheinberg IH, Jaffe ME, Sternlieb I. The use of trientine in preventing the effects of interrupting penicillamine therapy in Wilson's disease. N Engl J Med. 1987;317(4):209–13.
16. Walshe JM. The management of Wilson's disease with trienthylene tetramine 2HC1 (Trien 2HC1). Prog Clin Biol Res. 1979;34:271–80.
17. Saito T. Presenting symptoms and natural history of Wilson disease. Eur J Pediatr. 1987;146(3):261–5.
18. Saito H, et al. Triethylene-tetramine (trien) therapy for Wilson's disease. Tohoku J Exp Med. 1991;164(1):29–35.
19. Santos Silva EE, et al. Successful medical treatment of severely decompensated Wilson disease. J Pediatr. 1996;128(2):285–7.
20. European Association for Study of, L. EASL Clinical Practice Guidelines: Wilson's disease. J Hepatol. 2012;56(3):671–85.
21. Perry AR, et al. Acquired sideroblastic anaemia induced by a copper-chelating agent. Int J Hematol. 1996;64(1):69–72.
22. Condamine L, et al. Acquired sideroblastic anaemia during treatment of Wilson's disease with triethylene tetramine dihydrochloride. Br J Haematol. 1993;83(1):166–8.
23. Shiono Y, et al. Ultrastructural identification of iron and copper accumulation in the liver of a male patient with Wilson disease. Med Electron Microsc. 2001;34(1):54–60.
24. Brewer GJ, et al. Treatment of Wilson's disease with zinc: XV long-term follow-up studies. J Lab Clin Med. 1998;132(4):264–78.
25. Hoogenraad TU, Van Hattum J, Van den Hamer CJ. Management of Wilson's disease with zinc sulphate. Experience in a series of 27 patients. J Neurol Sci. 1987;77(2–3):137–46.

26. Hoogenraad TU. Zinc treatment of Wilson's disease. J Lab Clin Med. 1998;132(4):240–1.
27. Lee VD, Northup PG, Berg CL. Resolution of decompensated cirrhosis from Wilson's disease with zinc monotherapy: a potential therapeutic option? Clin Gastroenterol Hepatol. 2006;4(8):1069–71.
28. Yuzbasiyan-Gurkan V, et al. Treatment of Wilson's disease with zinc: X. Intestinal metallothionein induction. J Lab Clin Med. 1992;120(3):380–6.
29. Sturniolo GC, et al. Zinc therapy increases duodenal concentrations of metallothionein and iron in Wilson's disease patients. Am J Gastroenterol. 1999;94(2):334–8.
30. Brewer GJ, et al. Oral zinc therapy for Wilson's disease. Ann Intern Med. 1983;99(3):314–9.
31. Anderson LA, Hakojarvi SL, Boudreaux SK. Zinc acetate treatment in Wilson's disease. Ann Pharmacother. 1998;32(1):78–87.
32. Najda J, Stella-Holowiecka B, Machalski M. Low-dose zinc administration as an effective Wilson's disease treatment. Biol Trace Elem Res. 2001;80(3):281–4.
33. Huang CC, Chu NS. Wilson's disease: resolution of MRI lesions following long-term oral zinc therapy. Acta Neurol Scand. 1996;93(2–3):215–8.
34. Brewer GJ, et al. Treatment of Wilson's disease with zinc. XIII: therapy with zinc in presymptomatic patients from the time of diagnosis. J Lab Clin Med. 1994;123(6):849–58.
35. Milanino R, et al. Oral zinc as initial therapy in Wilson's disease: two years of continuous treatment in a 10-year-old child. Acta Paediatr. 1992;81(2):163–6.
36. Veen C, van den Hamer CJ, de Leeuw PW. Zinc sulphate therapy for Wilson's disease after acute deterioration during treatment with low-dose D-penicillamine. J Intern Med. 1991;229(6):549–52.
37. Rossaro L, et al. Zinc therapy in Wilson's disease: observations in five patients. Am J Gastroenterol. 1990;85(6):665–8.
38. Marcellini M, et al. Treatment of Wilson's disease with zinc from the time of diagnosis in pediatric patients: a single-hospital, 10-year follow-up study. J Lab Clin Med. 2005;145(3):139–43.
39. Linn FH, et al. Long-term exclusive zinc monotherapy in symptomatic Wilson disease: experience in 17 patients. Hepatology. 2009;50(5):1442–52.
40. Walshe JM, Munro NA. Zinc-induced deterioration in Wilson's disease aborted by treatment with penicillamine, dimercaprol, and a novel zero copper diet. Arch Neurol. 1995;52(1):10–1.

41. Lang CJ, et al. Fatal deterioration of Wilson's disease after institution of oral zinc therapy. Arch Neurol. 1993;50(10):1007–8.
42. Czlonkowska A, et al. Wilson's disease-cause of mortality in 164 patients during 1992-2003 observation period. J Neurol. 2005;252(6):698–703.
43. Roberts EA, Schilsky ML, American D, Association for Study of Liver. Diagnosis and treatment of Wilson disease: an update. Hepatology. 2008;47(6):2089–111.
44. Walshe JM, Yealland M. Chelation treatment of neurological Wilson's disease. Q J Med. 1993;86(3):197–204.
45. Pecoud A, Donzel P, Schelling JL. Effect of foodstuffs on the absorption of zinc sulfate. Clin Pharmacol Ther. 1975;17(4):469–74.
46. Hill GM, et al. Treatment of Wilson's disease with zinc. I. Oral zinc therapy regimens. Hepatology. 1987;7(3):522–8.
47. Dhawan A, et al. Wilson's disease in children: 37-year experience and revised King's score for liver transplantation. Liver Transpl. 2005;11(4):441–8.
48. Askari FK, et al. Treatment of Wilson's disease with zinc. XVIII. Initial treatment of the hepatic decompensation presentation with trientine and zinc. J Lab Clin Med. 2003;142(6):385–90.
49. Khanna A, et al. Liver transplantation for metabolic liver diseases. Surg Clin North Am. 1999;79(1):153–62. ix
50. Guarino M, et al. No neurological improvement after liver transplantation for Wilson's disease. Acta Neurol Scand. 1995;92(5):405–8.
51. Bellary S, Hassanein T, Van Thiel DH. Liver transplantation for Wilson's disease. J Hepatol. 1995;23(4):373–81.
52. Schilsky ML, Scheinberg IH, Sternlieb I. Liver transplantation for Wilson's disease: indications and outcome. Hepatology. 1994;19(3):583–7.
53. Schumacher G, et al. Liver transplantation: treatment of choice for hepatic and neurological manifestation of Wilson's disease. Clin Transpl. 1997;11(3):217–24.
54. Emre S, et al. Orthotopic liver transplantation for Wilson's disease: a single-center experience. Transplantation. 2001;72(7):1232–6.
55. Groth CG, et al. Metabolic effects of hepatic replacement in Wilson's disease. Transplant Proc. 1973;5(1):829–33.
56. Eghtesad B, et al. Liver transplantation for Wilson's disease: a single-center experience. Liver Transpl Surg. 1999;5(6):467–74.
57. Kassam N, et al. Liver transplantation for neuropsychiatric Wilson disease. Can J Gastroenterol. 1998;12(1):65–8.

58. Brewer GJ, et al. Treatment of Wilson's disease with tetrathiomolybdate: V. Control of free copper by tetrathiomolybdate and a comparison with trientine. Transl Res. 2009;154(2):70–7.
59. Senzolo M, et al. Different neurological outcome of liver transplantation for Wilson's disease in two homozygotic twins. Clin Neurol Neurosurg. 2007;109(1):71–5.
60. Barik A, et al. Evaluation of a new copper(II)-curcumin complex as superoxide dismutase mimic and its free radical reactions. Free Radic Biol Med. 2005;39(6):811–22.
61. van den Berghe PV, et al. Reduced expression of ATP7B affected by Wilson disease-causing mutations is rescued by pharmacological folding chaperones 4-phenylbutyrate and curcumin. Hepatology. 2009;50(6):1783–95.
62. Sinha S, et al. Is low serum tocopherol in Wilson's disease a significant symptom? J Neurol Sci. 2005;228(2):121–3.
63. Wang Y, et al. Clinical efficacy and safety of Chinese herbal medicine for Wilson's disease: a systematic review of 9 randomized controlled trials. Complement Ther Med. 2012;20(3):143–54.
64. Weiss KH, et al. Bis-choline tetrathiomolybdate in patients with Wilson's disease: an open-label, multicentre, phase 2 study. Lancet Gastroenterol Hepatol. 2017; 2(12):869–76
65. Schilsky MAF, Ferenci P, Ala A, Czlonkowska A, Nicholl D, Bronstein J, Bega D, Weiss KH. An ongoing extension of a phase 2 study of WTX-101 in newly diagnosed Wilson disease patients. Hepatology. 2017;66(S1):429A.
66. Ala A, Aliu E, Schilsky ML. Prospective pilot study of a single daily dosage of trientine for the treatment of Wilson disease. Dig Dis Sci. 2015;60(5):1433–9.

Chapter 4
Dietary Copper and Diet Issues for Patients with Wilson Disease

Anne Marie Rivard

Copper in Human Nutrition

Roles of Copper and Food Sources

Copper is a mineral critical to human health. It is an essential component of copper-dependent metalloenzymes which play roles in energy production, connective tissue formation, iron metabolism, central nervous system function, melanin formation, antioxidant functions, and regulation of gene expression [1]. The recommended dietary allowance (RDA) for copper for adults is 0.9 mg/day (900 μg/day) with median copper intake from foods in the United States of 1.0– mg/day as seen in the US National Health and Nutrition Examination Survey [2]. Any excess of copper ingested above the body's daily need will be excreted through the biliary system. Absorption

A. M. Rivard
Department of Food and Nutrition, Yale New Haven Hospital, New Haven, CT, USA
e-mail: annemarie.rivard@ynhh.org

M. L. Schilsky (ed.), *Management of Wilson Disease*, Clinical Gastroenterology, https://doi.org/10.1007/978-3-319-91527-2_4

of copper occurs in the small intestine, and the percent of copper absorbed declines with increasing daily intake. For example, more than 50% is absorbed when intake is <1 mg per day, whereas absorption is only 20% when intake rises above 5 mg per day. With the abovementioned median US copper intake, roughly 35% dietary copper absorption can be assumed [2]. For patients diagnosed with WD, the inability to excrete excess copper leads to a buildup throughout body tissues, and consequently, the sequelae of organ damage can then later occur.

Copper is found in a wide variety of foods. It is challenging to assign foods a "label," i.e., high copper versus low copper as the copper content of foods may vary depending on numerous factors, not all of which have been identified. It was proposed that copper content of soil may influence the mineral content of the plant, yet studies have not supported this theory [3]. In his 2016 article in the Journal of Food Composition and Analysis, Robin J Marles, a Canadian senior scientific advisor concludes that recent popular press reports noting declining mineral content of foods related to agricultural depletion of mineral content of soil can be explained simply by natural variation in the growing process [4]. The factors that affect this variation are not yet known. It was proposed that ripeness may affect the mineral content of foods, but there are few data to support this. For many years, researchers have studied the mineral content of foods, dating back as early as 1929. Lindow et al. published a study which identified the highest copper containing foods as liver, oysters, cocoa, nuts, dried legumes, cereals, dried fruits, poultry, fish, green legumes, roots, leafy vegetables, fresh fruits, and non-leafy vegetables [5]. Though the exact number of milligrams of copper found in these foods has changed over the years, even today these remain some of the top copper-dense foods. When searching the USDA food nutrient database for the copper content of specific foods, the foods with the highest amount of copper include liver, seaweed, sesame seeds, oysters, sweetbread, soy flour, cocoa, soy beans, cashews, mixed nuts, lentils, and sunflower seeds [6]. These are not the only foods that contain copper. The vast majority of foods within our food system contain some amount of copper, the amount varying greatly depending on portion size. In the USDA nutrient list, approximately 3% of foods or only 9.5 of the 293 pages of provided content have foods with zero copper content. The remaining 97% of foods within our food system have some copper content. Since dietary copper cannot be completely avoided, it is challenging for patients with WD to determine their optimal diet.

Copper Through the Life Span

Newborns

As WD is a genetic disorder, it is present in infancy. Even so, up until recently it was rare for young children to be tested and diagnosed as they did not show symptoms prompting testing. With genetic testing being much more common today, some individuals with this disorder are being diagnosed earlier in life. There is little research to date on the dynamics of copper intake and absorption in infants with WD, and therefore, very few recommendations on diet for these young individuals. There is no recommended level of copper intake for this group; rather, an adequate intake (AI) level of 0.2 mg/day is set for infants that reflects the observed mean copper intake of infants fed principally human milk [2]. For the first 4–6 months of life for all infants, the main source of nutrition should be breastmilk or an infant formula to ensure adequate nutrient intake during this critical period of growth. The copper content of human milk is found to be on average 0.36 mg/L [7], though the actual content appears to change significantly throughout the course of lactation, being highest within the first few weeks after birth (0.452 mg/L), decreasing by month 4 (0.298 mg/L), and then rising again by month 9 (0.556 mg/L) [8]. Entry of copper in to breastmilk appears to be via active transport, meaning copper content of breastmilk is independent of maternal copper status. Studies have confirmed that maternal copper status does not influence copper content of breastmilk. The changes in copper concentration of breastmilk throughout the lactation period as noted above will occur regardless of the mother's diet [9]. Regardless of point in lactation, cow's milk as compared to human milk is significantly lower in copper at 0.06–0.09 mg/L [2]. Although cow's milk would provide much less copper to an infant, it is an otherwise nutritionally inadequate option for infants in general and should not be introduced prior to 12 months of age. Cow's milk is low in iron content, presenting a significant risk of anemia for infants. Cow's milk is also much higher in calcium and casein than breast milk, leading to a high renal solute load. The renal solute load refers to the waste substances of both dietary and endogenous origin that require excretion by the kidneys. The high solute load from the casein content of cow's milk requires increased amounts of water for excretion through the kidneys and therefore can increase the risk of dehydration in an infant [10]. For these reasons and more, cow's milk should not be given to children under 1 year of age. If breastmilk is not an option, infant formulas are recommended. These contain the proper concentration of nutrients and mimic breastmilk as closely as possible to provide ideal nutrition. The copper content of most infant formulas is comparable to breastmilk [7], with most standard commercially available brands in the United States providing 0.4–0.6 mg/L. Based on these numbers, either breastmilk or infant formulas appear to be appropriate choices for infants with WD, with further research being needed on the impact of dietary copper intake in the first year of life in these individuals.

Toddlers and Children

As children begin to take table food and wean away from breastmilk and/or infant formula around 4–6 months, their copper intake begins to vary based on their dietary intake. A recommended dietary allowance (RDA) has been set for this group for the amount of copper that needs to be ingested to meet the needs of 97.5% of this population. The RDA for copper intake for children 1–3 years old is 0.34 mg/day, children 4–8 years old is 0.44 mg/day, 9–13 years old is 0.7 mg/day, and children 14–18 years old is 0.89 mg/day [2]. As stated previously, cow's milk is quite low in copper content and provides a significant portion of calories for the growing toddler (>1 year of age) and young children. It is helpful to introduce a wide variety of foods in the first years of life to present various tastes to a developing palate. This may also play a role in reducing risk of developing food allergies, though the recommendations in this field continue to change with ongoing research [11]. There is no reason to overly restrict a child's diet, especially since the portions consumed are quite small. That being said, it might be helpful to steer intake toward lower copper foods to help develop taste preferences for these foods, making diet later in life feel less restrictive. Parents should be encouraged to offer all foods to their child while guiding them to base their daily intake around lower copper foods choices which will be discussed later in the chapter.

Dietary Modifications in Wilson Disease

Food

Copper is present in a wide variety of foods within our food system. For this reason, a true low-copper diet can be challenging to follow and still maintain nutritional adequacy. At present, there is no data on the effect of dietary copper intake on WD progression and therefore no research to support an overly restrictive diet in patients on effective medical therapy. Information currently available to patients ranges from recommendations for very low-copper diets to no dietary restrictions at all [12]. Most commonly, it is suggested that individuals with WD limit dietary copper intake to 1 mg or less per day, which is comparable to the RDA. The American Association for the Study of Liver Diseases (AASLD) recommends that "patients should avoid intake of foods and water with high concentrations of copper, especially in the first year of treatment"[13]. This broad variability in recommendations presents challenges when educating a newly diagnosed WD patient. Do they need to follow a low-copper diet? What foods should be eliminated? The needle of consensus on this topic seems to be moving slowly toward less restrictive diets in WD patients with stable disease on therapy.

As noted previously, on average approximately 35% of copper from food is absorbed. Even consuming only foods considered higher in copper, very large quantities would be needed for the amount of copper absorbed to be clinically significant. Additionally, restricting copper intake to a very low-copper diet will actually cause an increase in the percent of copper absorbed from foods, therefore defeating the purpose of trying to decrease copper intake. Presently, there is minimal evidence-based research which supports overly restrictive diets.

Questions remain regarding the effects of omnivorous diets versus vegetarian/vegan diets. While the plant-based foods consumed through a vegan diet may provide roughly twice the copper content of an omnivorous diet, the presence of fiber and phytates within these foods makes the copper less bioavailable [14]. Therefore, a vegetarian or vegan diet is not contraindicated for a WD patient. Although these points minimize the need for a very restrictive diet, diet and nutrition still play a role within management of WD. Some foods have such a significantly elevated copper content that even with an assumed 35% absorption, copper intake would be over 1 mg per serving. These foods include liver (6–13 mg per average serving) and most shellfish (5 mg per average serving, excluding scallops). These foods should be avoided during the first year of treatment and then included in the diet only on rare occasions thereafter.

While a true dietary restriction is not necessary based on current evidence, patients should still be provided with nutritional counseling. In practice, patients view diet as an area in which they have control and are often looking for guidance on what foods to eat. While diet alone cannot manage WD, when included with medical therapy, it can be an integral part of overall management. It may not be appropriate for all individuals, yet in practice there is found to be large subset of patients who benefit from clear and specific guidelines on beneficial food choices. Diet advice can be provided in a clear and nutritionally sound fashion. These patients often do their own research and end up overly restricting foods based on the varying evidence they find online. They benefit from specific information from a nutrition professional on the copper content of foods with guidelines laid out on what foods to enjoy, what foods to moderate and what foods to minimize. When presenting this information, it is important to do it in a one-on-one setting with a registered dietitian (RD) who assesses the individual's level of understanding and tailors education accordingly. Nutritional consultation is also recommended to provide guidance to patients on how to best maintain an optimal nutritional status as excess intake, weight gain, and elevated cholesterol panels can all contribute to long-term liver dysfunction in a group of patients that is already at risk for liver compromise due to their underlying disease.

The table below (Table 4.1) provides recommended dietary intake guidelines to patients based on copper content of foods. It should be noted that foods are divided into three categories: low-copper foods, moderate-copper foods, and high-copper foods. Those low in copper provide less than 0.08 mg of copper per average serving and do not pose a significant copper burden when consumed. Moderate-copper foods provide up to 0.2 mg of copper per serving and, if consumed in larger portions, could provide a significant amount of copper. For that reason, the portion size of these foods should be monitored, but they do not need to be avoided altogether. High-copper foods are those that have more than 0.2 mg per serving. The copper content of these foods can add up quickly, and they should be consumed less frequently (weekly to monthly).

Table 4.1 Copper content of selected foods according to data from the USDA food nutrient database

	Low-copper foods (< 0.08 mg/serving) ***Enjoy these foods***	**Moderate-copper foods (0.08 mg–0.2 mg/serving)** ***Monitor portions of these foods***	**High-copper foods (> 0.2 mg/serving)** ***Choose these foods less frequently***
Bread and grains	White bread, pasta, rice Cream of wheat Cereals such as Cheerios, Kix, Cinnamon Toast Crunch, Rice Krispies	Wheat bread (1 slice) Wheat spaghetti (½ cup) Whole wheat crackers (6) Brown or wild rice (½ cup) Instant or old-fashioned oatmeal (1 cup) Shredded wheat (1 cup) Canned beans, chickpeas (½ cup) Quinoa, barley, millet (½ cup cooked) Wheat germ (3 tablespoons)	Dried beans, peas, lentils Soy flour Soy grits Bran cereals

Dairy	Cow's milk Almond milk (non-chocolate flavored) Cheese, cottage cheese Yogurt Frozen yogurt, ice creams (non-chocolate flavored)	Chocolate cow's milk (1 cup) Chocolate almond milk (1 cup) Frozen yogurts, ice creams (chocolate flavored) (½ cup) Hot cocoa mix (3 tsp)	Soy milk Vitamin-fortified nutrition shakes (Boost, Ensure, Glucerna, Carnation Instant Breakfast, etc.)
Sweets	Jams, jellies Candies made with allowed ingredients Carob Flavoring extracts Maple syrup	Gummi bears (1.5 oz) Molasses (1 tablespoon) Milk chocolate (1.5 oz)	Desserts or candy that contain nuts, dark chocolate, or cocoa Trail mix

(continued)

TABLE 4.1 (continued)

	Low-copper foods (< 0.08 mg/serving) *Enjoy these foods*	**Moderate-copper foods (0.08 mg–0.2 mg/serving)** *Monitor portions of these foods*	**High-copper foods (> 0.2 mg/serving)** *Choose these foods less frequently*
Vegetables	Most vegetables (cucumber, green beans, Brussels sprouts, celery, eggplant, lettuce, broccoli, cauliflower, collard greens, onions, green peppers, fresh tomatoes, fresh spinach, cabbage, carrots, jicama, bok choy, mixed frozen vegetables) Boxed mashed potatoes Shiitake and enoki mushrooms	Bean sprouts (1 cup) Cooked spinach, kale, broccoli rabe or okra (½ cup) Tomato juice, canned tomato products including spaghetti sauce (½ cup) Asparagus, green peas, all squash varieties, artichokes (½ cup) Pumpkin (3/4 cup) Potato without skin (1 med) Sauerkraut (½ cup) Turnips, parsnips (1 cup) Mushrooms (other than two noted low copper) (½ cup)	Vegetable juice Lima beans Sweet potato Potatoes with skin

Fruits	Most fruits (apples, strawberries, melons, applesauce, blueberries, cherries, grapefruit, oranges, peaches, watermelon, plums, canned fruit) Dried cranberries (up to ¾ cup) Cranberry, apple, or grape juice	Mango (½ each) Pear, banana, kiwi, nectarine (1) Pineapple (1 cup) Raspberries, blackberries, grapes (½ cup) Prune, orange, grapefruit, pineapple juice (1 cup) Avocado (½ each)	Dried fruits (except dried cranberries)
Protein	Most fish (tuna, orange roughy, halibut, trout, haddock, flounder, sole, cod) Scallops Eggs White meat turkey and chicken All beef hotdogs Bacon	Beef (includes steak, hamburger) (3 oz) Pork (includes ham) (3 oz) Dark meat turkey (3 oz) Dark meat chicken (3 oz) Peanut butter (2 Tbsp.) Shrimp (4 large) Mussels (3 oz) Swordfish or salmon (3 oz) Hummus (1 tablespoon)	Organ meat (liver, kidney, brain, heart) Lamb lobster, oysters, crab, clams, squid Quail, duck, and goose Hotdogs with pork, turkey, or chicken Soy protein, soy beans, tofu Nuts and seeds

(continued)

TABLE 4.1 (continued)

	Low-copper foods (< 0.08 mg/serving) ***Enjoy these foods***	**Moderate-copper foods (0.08 mg–0.2 mg/serving)** ***Monitor portions of these foods***	**High-copper foods (> 0.2 mg/serving)** ***Choose these foods less frequently***
Fats, oils, condiments	Butter, margarine Cream, nondairy creamer Mayonnaise, sour cream Oils, salad dressings Olives, pickles		
Beverages	Coffee, tea Fruit juices, fruit-flavored beverages Lemonade Carbonated beverages		Mineral water (like Perrier or Pellegrino)

Water

Copper content of drinking water can vary, often depending on the plumbing which brings water to the tap. Copper in drinking water will be in an inorganic form, meaning it is in metal salt-based form as opposed to the carbon-based organic form found naturally in foods. Copper is often used in pipes and other building materials, and over time, the copper from the pipes can leach into water. Studies have found the copper content of water varying from <0.005 mg/L to as high as 30 mg/L [15] due to varying infrastructure. Copper content of municipal water sources are monitored and fall under the Lead and Copper Rule (LCR) published by the Environmental Protection Agency (EPA) in 1991. This requires utility companies to monitor the copper content of water at the customer tap level. If levels of copper exceed 1.3 ppm in >10% of taps surveyed, action must be taken to lower copper content of the water by addressing infrastructure issues [16]. When the water source is a private well, there could be varying levels of copper in the water based on the ground source. It is recommended that all patients, regardless of water source, have their water checked for mineral content upon initial diagnosis. Water with a copper content over 0.1 mg/L is considered elevated for this patient population, and steps should be taken to reduce copper content of water. Copper levels are highest when taps are first turned on if water has been sitting in contact with copper containing plumbing. Most of the older copper plumbing has surfaces that are oxidized and therefore will leach less copper and do not have to be replaced for patients with WD. However, copper content decreases considerably as the water runs, and individuals with WD should be encouraged to use cold tap water and allow the tap to run for a short period of time until the water is cool before collecting water for cooking or drinking. Additionally, home water filters can be used to safely further decrease the copper content of tap water. It is important that the replaceable filters from these units be changed at the recommended intervals per the manufacturer's guidelines to ensure proper removal of copper. At this time, there are no published data regarding the efficacy of specific brands of filters, so no specific recommendations can be provided at this time.

Cooking Methods

Copper cookware, including pots, pans, utensils, and mugs, are marketed as excellent cooking vessels with the ability to change temperature quickly while evenly spreading out heat. Over time, they can leach some of their copper content into foods, especially when more acidic foods such as tomatoes are added to the cooking vessel. This will increase the copper content of food without increasing nutritional value. Therefore, all individuals with WD should be encouraged to avoid copper containing cooking and dining utensils.

Nutritional Supplements

The nutritional supplement industry is a multi-billion-dollar industry that pervades many aspects of everyday life. From well-meaning friends and family, to television personalities and celebrities, the average individual is presented with supplement marketing on a regular basis. It is important that patients understand the distinction between prescription medications and dietary supplements; dietary supplements do not require proof of safety or efficacy before being brought to market. For this reason, one cannot be 100% sure that what is represented on the label of a supplement is actually contained in that product. Patients should be encouraged to research the safety and efficacy of a product with their practitioner before use, ideally seeking out supplements that are certified by independent labs such as US Pharmacopeia (USP) dietary supplement verification program. Copper is present in many supplements from standard multivitamins (Centrum®- 1 mg copper per serving) to supplements marketed to help with liver function, depression, infertility, and many other conditions. These supplements often contain approximately 2 mg copper per serving, well above the RDA. They are present in an inorganic salt form, and it is unclear how much is actually absorbed. As most individuals can get the micronutrients they need from a well-balanced diet, it is recommended that all supplemental copper be avoided by individuals with WD to eliminate this unnecessary source of copper ingestion.

Oral liquid nutritional supplements are another source of inorganic copper in the diet. These drinks (such as Ensure®, Boost®, and Carnation Breakfast Essentials®) are marketed to individuals with poor appetite and a busy schedule or for anyone that needs ready-to-go nutrition. As these are made to supplement the diet of individuals who are assumed to have inadequate intake, these are fortified with a wide range of vitamins and minerals, including copper. These mineral-fortified supplements should be avoided for individuals with WD, as should supplements with pea protein as their main source of protein due to the high-copper content of peas. If individuals require a concentrated source of nutrition in shake format, SlimFast® is one option (180 calories and 10 grams protein per bottle) as it is not fortified with copper and uses milk protein as its base. Individuals can also make their own shakes and smoothies using low-copper food including milk, fruit, yogurt, and with whey-based protein powder or powdered egg whites as indicated. Individuals are encouraged to meet with a Registered Dietitian to determine their nutritional requirements.

Special Considerations

Liver Disease

Due to the inability to excrete excess copper in WD, copper deposition may occur throughout the body, most notably in the liver. If left untreated, this can progress to cirrhosis, which presents a unique set of nutritional considerations. Patients with cirrhosis may be hypermetabolic, requiring increased calories and protein to maintain nutritional homeostasis. This often coincides with a decrease in appetite and intake and can lead very quickly to malnutrition. Approximately 50–90% of patients with cirrhosis have been found to have protein calorie malnutrition [17]. This is concerning, in that poor nutritional status is associated with increased mortality and other complications [17]. Early nutrition intervention can prevent nutritional decline and maintain robust nutritional status throughout the course of cirrhosis. Calorie and protein needs for patients with cirrhosis are elevated to 35–40 kcals/kg ideal body weight and 1.0–1.5 g protein/kg ideal body weight [17]. Individuals with cirrhosis are encouraged to have small, frequent, balanced meals with encouragement of a bedtime snack to prevent nocturnal hypoglycemia and improve lean body mass [18]. These individuals are also at increased risk for development of ascites and are encouraged to choose foods in their diet that are lower in sodium such that their daily intake is 2 grams or less. Patients are discouraged from adding salt to their foods and encouraged to read labels to monitor sodium content. It is recommended that they avoid alcohol intake to prevent further hepatic compromise. They should seek out a consultation with an RD to evaluate their diet and optimize intake.

Neurological Involvement

Dysphagia

If WD progresses such that there is neurological impairment, an individual's ability to safely swallow must be evaluated. All patients with suspected neurological involvement should have a consultation with a speech language pathologist (SLP) to determine optimal diet consistency. If any dysphagia is noted, thickened liquids and altered diet consistencies may be required. There are many commercially available thickening agents which use cornstarch as a base and can safely thicken food. Individuals should continue to work with an SLP throughout the course of their treatment as their swallowing capabilities may change. If it is deemed unsafe for patients to swallow any consistency, alternative nutrition support may be needed, and this is discussed next. In patients who were unable to swallow or had limitations and who improve with therapy, repeat testing for swallowing under observation by a professional is recommended prior to restarting a standard diet.

Nutrition Support

Individuals with a compromised ability to swallow due to neurological involvement in their WD may require tube feeding to maintain nutritional status while lowering risk of aspiration. The challenge lies in crafting the optimal nutrition support regimen. Most commercially available tube feeding preparations have added copper and provide close to 3 mg of copper per day, far beyond the recommended ~1 mg per day for WD patients. As this is mostly in an inorganic form, absorption may differ from the absorption of organic copper in food, though data in humans is not available to say conclusively at this time. Various recipes exist to make homemade low-copper tube feeding using ingredients such as evaporated whole milk, baby food, and protein powders. Patients should work closely with an RD when mixing homemade enteral formulas. Aseptic techniques must be used while mixing and ingredients and recipes should be evaluated by an RD to ensure nutritional adequacy.

Another option is to use a concentrated commercially available formula (such as TwoCal® by Abbott) but meet only approximately 50% of calorie needs with this formula. The remaining 50% of calorie needs can be met using evaporated whole milk and a carbohydrate modular product. The below recipe (Table 4.2) provides 2294 calories and 87.8 grams protein with approximately 48% of calories coming from carbohydrate, 16% from protein, and 36% from fat,

TABLE 4.2 Low-copper tube feed recipe using standard adult formula as a base

Product	**Quantity**	**Kcals**	**Carbohydrates (grams)**	**Protein (grams)**	**Fat (grams)**	**Volume (milliliters)**	**Free water (milliliters)**	**Copper (milligrams)**
TwoCal	Two cans (16 oz total)	950	103.6	39.8	43	474	332	1
Evaporated whole milk	Two cans (48 oz total)	960	72	48	48	708	560	0.121
PolyCal	100 grams	384	96	0	0	0	0	0
Water	318 ml	0	0	0	0	318	318	0
		2294	271.6	87.8	91	1500	1210	1.121

TABLE 4.3 Low-copper tube feed option using standard pediatric formula

	Calories	CHO	Pro	Fat	Copper	Volume
6.5 cans Pediasure 1.5®	2275	247	91	104	1.3	1540

appropriate for most adults with average nutritional needs. This recipe can be further modified under the guidance of an RD to ensure appropriate macronutrient and micronutrient intake on a patient-specific basis. The amount of PolyCal® can be adjusted (carbohydrate modular), a protein modular can be added (such as BeneProtein®), or a combined fat and carbohydrate modular may be added (DuoCal®) to optimize the formula as needed. Additionally, the amount of free water added can be adjusted to ensure fluid needs are met.

Commercially prepared formulas for the pediatric population may also present an option for adult patients needing lower copper formulations. Their mineral content is lower to meet the RDA's of younger children but in larger volumes can still provide nutritionally adequate options for adults. Pediasure 1.5® is a calorically dense formula that only has 0.2 mg of copper per 8 oz can. Using 6 ½ cans per day would provide the nutritional equivalent of a homemade formula in a ready-to-feed formulation (Table 4.3). Insurance coverage, patient support system, home environment, and patient tolerance all must be taken in to consideration when choosing an appropriate enteral nutrition regimen.

Resources

One-on-One RD Assistance

Living with WD can be a challenging course to navigate alone. Patients are encouraged to reach out to all members of their care team and ensure they have adequate support to optimize their lifestyle. An RD is an integral member of that team. Every individual has unique diet and lifestyle factors which cannot be captured in a chart format. For that reason, all patients should be encouraged to meet one on one with a nutrition professional to plan their optimal diet. Patients can visit http://www.eatright.org/find-an-expert to find a nutrition professional in their area. Or they can call their local hospital to inquire about outpatient nutrition services. Patients are encouraged to check with their insurance when scheduling such visits to understand their coverage and out of pocket costs. Patients can also ask if there is an RD working with their gastroenterologist or hepatologist.

USDA Food/Nutrient Database

The USDA, through its Nutrient Data Laboratory, keeps an online record of the nutrient content of most standard foods, found at https://ndb.nal.usda.gov/ndb/ [19]. This is kept up to date and includes data on the micronutrient content of foods, including copper content. As noted below (Fig. 4.1), when searching for copper content of foods, ensure the data source is "standard reference" as opposed to "branded food products" to ensure there is data on copper content.

Once the desired food is found in the database, select "Full Report" to see the copper content (Fig. 4.2).

After scrolling down, the copper content will be listed under the "minerals" section, and content for the selected food is listed in milligrams for the selected portion size (Fig. 4.3).

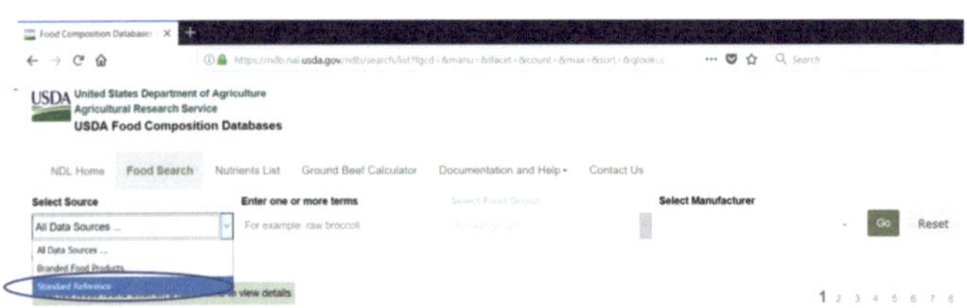

FIG. 4.1 Choosing "standard reference" in the USDA food composition database, found at https://ndb.nal.usda.gov/ndb/search/list

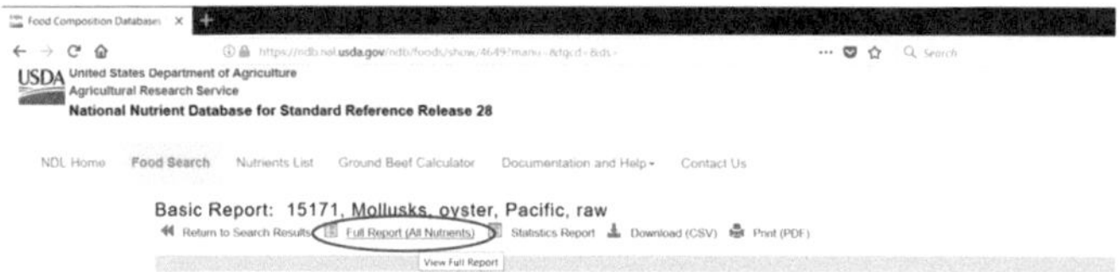

FIG. 4.2 Choosing "full report" in the USDA food composition database, found at https://ndb.nal.usda.gov/ndb/search/list

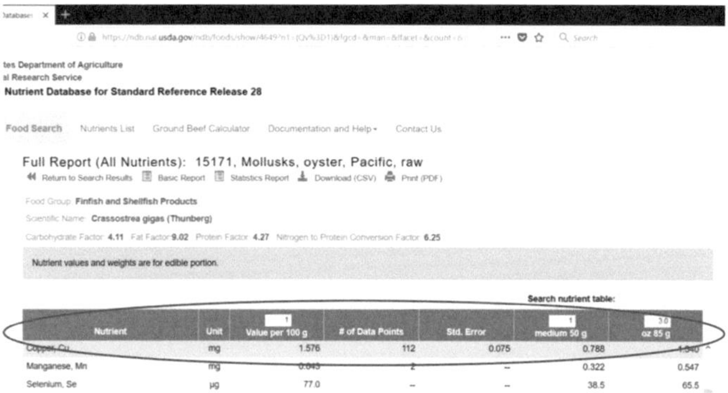

FIG. 4.3 Finding copper content in the USDA food composition database, found at https://ndb.nal.usda.gov/ndb/search/list

This can be a useful tool for individuals who wish to understand the copper content of foods and find lower copper substitutes for commonly consumed foods.

Conclusion

There is still much to be learned about the connection between diet and WD. While we know that overly restrictive diets are likely unnecessary, as well as cumbersome and potentially nutritionally inadequate, nutrition has a central role in WD management. Diet is one important piece in the health maintenance for individuals with this diagnosis and can play a role in maintaining liver health as well. Further research is needed in many areas, including nutrition support regimens, nutrition management for infants with WD, dietary copper's impact on disease progression, and more.

References

1. Copper. http://lpi.oregonstate.edu/mic/minerals/copper
2. Press NA. Institute of Medicine (US) Panel on Micronutrients. Dietary Reference Intakes for Vitamin A, Vitamin K, Arsenic, Boron, Chromium, Copper, Iodine, Iron, Manganese, Molybdenum, Nickel, Silicon, Vanadium, and Zinc.; 2001. https://www.ncbi.nlm.nih.gov/books/NBK222312/
3. Badilla-Ohlbaum R, Ginocchio R, Rodriguez PH, Céspedes A. Relationship between soil copper content and copper content of selected crop plants in central Chile. Environ Toxicol Chem. 2001;20(12):2749–57. http://onlinelibrary.wiley.com/doi/10.1002/etc.5620201214/full
4. Marles RJ. Mineral nutrient composition of vegetables, fruits and grains: the context of reports of apparent historical declines. J Food Compos Anal. 2017;56:93–103. https://doi.org/10.1016/j.jfca.2016.11.012.
5. Lindow C, Elvehjem C, Peterson W. The copper content of plant and animal foods. J Biol Chem. 1929;82:465–71.
6. US Department of Agriculture, Agricultural Research Service, Nutrient Data Laboratory. USDA National Nutrient Database for Standard Reference, Release 28. Version Current: September 2015, slightly revised May 2016. https://ndb.nal.usda.gov/ndb/. Accessed 12 July 2017.
7. Khaghani S, Ezzatpanah H, Mazhari N, Givianrad MH, Mirmiranpour H, Sadrabadi FS. Zinc and copper concentrations in human milk and infant formulas. Iran J Pediatr. 2010;20(1):53–7.
8. Songul Yalcin S, Yalcin S, Ihsan Gucus A. Zinc and copper concentrations in breast milk during the first nine months of lactation: a longitudinal study. Pediatrics. 2015;135:S13–4. https://doi.org/10.1542/peds.2014.
9. Domellöf M, Lönnerdal B, Dewey KG, Cohen RJ, Hernell O. Iron , zinc , and copper concentrations in breast milk are independent of maternal mineral status. Am J Clin Nutr. 2004;79(1):1–3.

10. Ziegler EE. Adverse effects of cow's milk in infants. Nestle Nutr Workshop Ser Pediatr Program. 2007;60:185–99.
11. Fleischer DM, Sicherer S, TePas E. Introducing highly allergenic foods to infants and children. https://www.uptodate.com/contents/introducing-highly-allergenic-foods-to-infants-and-children#H2497362924. Published 2017. Accessed 12 July 2017.
12. Russell K, Gillanders LK, Orr DW, Plank LD. Dietary copper restriction in Wilson's disease. Eur J Clin Nutr. 2017;72:326. https://doi.org/10.1038/s41430-017-0002-0.
13. Roberts E, Schilsky M. Diagnosis and treatment of Wilson disease: an update. Hepatology. 2008;47:2089–111.
14. Bost M, Houdart S, Oberli M, Kalonji E, Huneau JF, Margaritis I. Dietary copper and human health: current evidence and unresolved issues. J Trace Elem Med Biol. 2016;35:107–15. https://doi.org/10.1016/j.jtemb.2016.02.006.
15. WHO. Copper in drinking-water. America (NY). 2011;3:23. doi:https://doi.org/10.1016/j.kjms.2011.05.002.
16. lead-and-copper-rule @ www.epa.gov
17. Cheung K, Lee SS, Raman M. Prevalence and mechanisms of malnutrition in patients with advanced liver disease, and nutrition management strategies. Clin Gastroenterol Hepatol. 2012;10(2):117–25. https://doi.org/10.1016/j.cgh.2011.08.016.
18. Tsien CD, Mccullough AJ, Dasarathy S. Late evening snack: exploiting a period of anabolic opportunity in cirrhosis. J Gastroenterol Hepatol. 2012;27(3):430–41. https://doi.org/10.1111/j.1440-1746.2011.06951.x.
19. US Department of Agriculture, Agricultural Research Service, Nutrient Data Laboratory. USDA National Nutrient Database for Standard Reference, Release 28. Version Current: September 2015. Internet: /nea/bhnrc/ndl

Chapter 5
Treating Other Symptoms of Wilson Disease: The Liver

Michelle Camarata and Michael L. Schilsky

Introduction

Symptoms of Wilson disease (WD) normally first present between the ages of 5 and 35 years old with liver-related symptoms occurring more frequently in younger patients and neurological symptoms occurring in patients presenting at an older age. Around 40–50% of WD patients will present with symptomatic liver dis-

M. Camarata
Department of Gastroenterology and Hepatology, Royal Surrey County Hospital, Guildford, Surrey, UK

Department of Clinical and Experimental Medicine, University of Surrey, Guildford, Surrey, UK

Department of Surgery, Section of Transplant and Immunology, Yale School of Medicine, New Haven, CT, USA
e-mail: michelle.camarata@yale.edu

M. L. Schilsky (✉)
Division of Digestive Diseases and Transplant and Immunology, Departments of Medicine and Surgery, Yale University, New Haven, CT, USA
e-mail: michael.schilsky@yale.edu

M. L. Schilsky (ed.), *Management of Wilson Disease*, Clinical Gastroenterology, https://doi.org/10.1007/978-3-319-91527-2_5

TABLE 5.1 Summary of clinical signs and symptoms and their medical treatment options

Clinical symptom/ sign	Treatment options
Jaundice (Advanced liver disease)	Decoppering therapy Low copper diet Avoidance of toxic liver injury (alcohol, liver toxic medications)
Varices	Nonselective beta-blockers (e.g., propranolol, nadolol) Endoscopic band ligation (esophageal) Sclerotherapy with glue (gastric) TIPS BRTO
Ascites	Salt restriction Diuretics Paracentesis TIPS or surgical shunt
Hepatic Encephalopathy	Lactulose Enemas (if oral route not possible) Nonabsorbed antibiotics (e.g., rifaximin, neomycin)

ease [12]. The severity of symptoms related to the liver in WD can be very variable and is related to the degree of inflammation and damage to the liver. The most common signs and symptoms of liver disease are yellowing of the skin (jaundice) and loss of appetite (anorexia) (37–44%), followed by fluid accumulation in the abdominal cavity (ascites) (23–26%) and enlargement of the liver and spleen (16–29%) [8, 17, 26]. Table 5.1 provides a summary of the clinical signs and symptoms that can present in patients with Wilson disease and their medical treatment options.

Asymptomatic or Mild Symptoms

Persistently abnormal liver blood tests, in particular liver transaminases (ALT and AST) can indicate hepatitis, which simply implies inflammation of the liver. At this early stage when there may only be abnormal lab tests and patients lack symptoms, the most common and only finding on physical examination might be a mildly enlarged liver. Asymptomatic WD patients with only a mild elevation of liver tests are reported to occur in about 18–25% of patients [8, 26]. Persistent liver inflammation can eventually result in scarring or fibrosis of the liver tissue. For the purposes of standardization, the degree of fibrosis present can be divided into stages. The last stage characterized by scarring and regenerative growth of remaining areas in response to injury to form nodules of the liver is called cirrhosis. Initially, cirrhosis can begin as compensated disease and sometimes can be clinically silent with few symptoms noted by patients. When the liver disease progresses, symptoms may include skin changes such as jaundice and icteric sclerae (yellowing of the white part of the eye) and spider nevi which are small spiderlike blood vessels that develop on the surface of the skin, commonly found on the face, neck, and upper part of the trunk and arms. Other symptoms may include easy bruising or bleeding (including nosebleeds or bleeding gums), red palms of the hand known as palmar erythema, and muscle wasting. Physical examination of the abdomen may also demonstrate an enlarged spleen.

Portal Hypertension

With progression of liver disease and cirrhosis, more serious symptoms can develop due to the increased resistance to the blood flowing through the liver causing a raised portal venous pressure which is the blood pressure in the hepatic vein. Raised portal venous pressure is termed portal hypertension. Measuring the hepatic venous pressure gradient (HVPG) is accepted as the gold standard for assessing the severity of portal hypertension [10]. It is determined by wedging a catheter in a hepatic vein to occlude it and measuring the pressure of the proximal static blood to calculate the wedged hepatic venous pressure (WHVP). The HVPG is the pressure gradient between the WHVP and the free hepatic venous pressure [10]. Portal hypertension is defined as an HVPG greater than or equal to 5 mm Hg and is clinically significant when the HVPG exceeds 10–12 mm Hg. Table 5.2 illustrates the complications that can occur as portal hypertension progresses.

Measuring the portal pressure is invasive and clinically impractical and therefore clinicians are more often guided by clinical signs and symptoms as well as imaging and endoscopic findings. For instance, new development of varices on endoscopic appearance indicates the recruitment of collateral vessels and increase in portal pressure.

Varices (Esophageal and Gastric)

A very serious complication of portal hypertension is bleeding from varices, abnormally enlarged veins (similar to varicose veins) that form within the lining of the esophagus or within the stomach and rarely in other places in the gut (see Figs. 5.1 and 5.2). They form because of the increased portal pressure that encourages the development of collateral blood flow around the liver. When enlarged, these varices can become fragile due to increased wall tension and can suddenly burst to cause serious, life-threatening bleeding.

In some patients with WD, bleeding from the varices may be the first presenting symptom of their disease. In others found to have cirrhosis, an upper endoscopy should be performed to screen for varices, and repeat testing (surveillance) performed on a yearly basis as varices will develop over time with disease progression. If larger varices are found on direct examination, medications such as nonselective beta-blockers (e.g., propranolol or nadolol) can also reduce portal pressure and thereby the blood flow running through the varices and decrease the risk of variceal bleeding [27]. Nonselective beta-blockers should be taken at the maximum tolerated dose and are adjusted based on pulse or blood pressure. Once a patient is committed to nonselective beta-blocker therapy, yearly endoscopic surveillance for varices may no longer be needed.

TABLE 5.2 Progression of liver disease and complications of portal hypertension. The diagram below indicates how portal pressures correlate with clinical findings and medical management of these. When medical management is not possible, liver transplant may be considered. The normal portal venous pressure measurement is <5 mm Hg. Complications arise when the portal pressure gradient exceeds 10–12 mmHg

Portal pressures (HVPG)	**1–5 mm Hg**	**6–10 mm Hg**	**10–12 mm Hg**	**>12 mm Hg**	**>20 mm Hg**

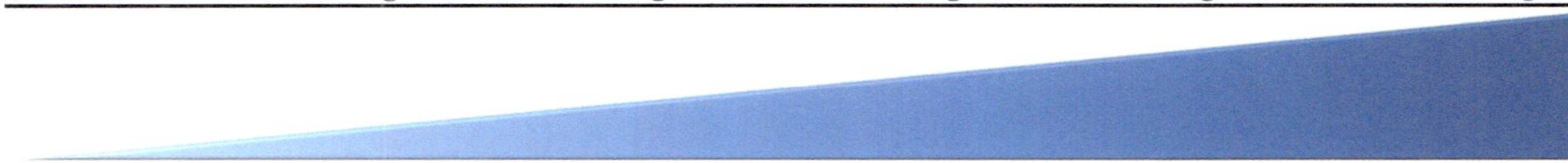

Clinical findings	*Chronic inflammation*	*Hepatic fibrosis* Splenomegaly	*Compensated cirrhosis* Development of collateral vessels	*Decompensated cirrhosis* Variceal bleeding Ascites Hepatic encephalopathy Jaundice	*Late (further) decompensation* Recurrent variceal hemorrhage Refractory ascites Recurrent hepatic encephalopathy Hepatorenal syndrome Jaundice

(continued)

Table 5.2 (continued)

Portal pressures (HVPG)	**1–5 mm Hg**	**6–10 mm Hg**	**10–12 mm Hg**	**>12 mm Hg**	**>20 mm Hg**
Management	Treat underlying cause	Endoscopic screening +/– Elective band ligation therapy Nonselective b-blockade	Endoscopic screening +/– Elective band ligation therapy Nonselective b-blockade	Emergency band ligation therapy TIPS Transplant evaluation Diuretics +/– paracentesis Lactulose +/– non-absorbed antibiotics	Emergency band ligation therapy TIPS Transplant evaluation Diuretics +/– paracentesis Lactulose +/– non-absorbed antibiotics

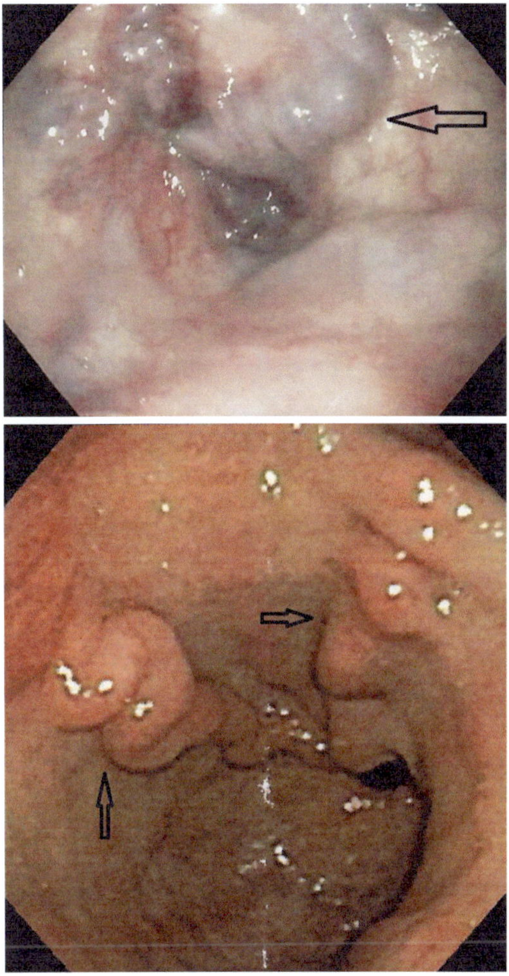

FIGURE 5.1 AND 5.2 Esophageal varices. Endoscopic view of esophageal varices. Figure 5.1: Prominent varix (arrow) in the distal esophagus just above the gastroesophageal junction (GOJ). Figure 5.2: Shown are multiple esophageal varices in the distal esophagus (arrows)

Direct measurement of the change in the portal pressure due to the medication is rarely performed. If nonselective beta-blockers are not tolerated, bleeding from esophageal varices can also be prevented by endoscopically placing rubber bands on the blood vessels to collapse them, a procedure known as variceal ligation (see Figs. 5.3 and 5.4). This ligation

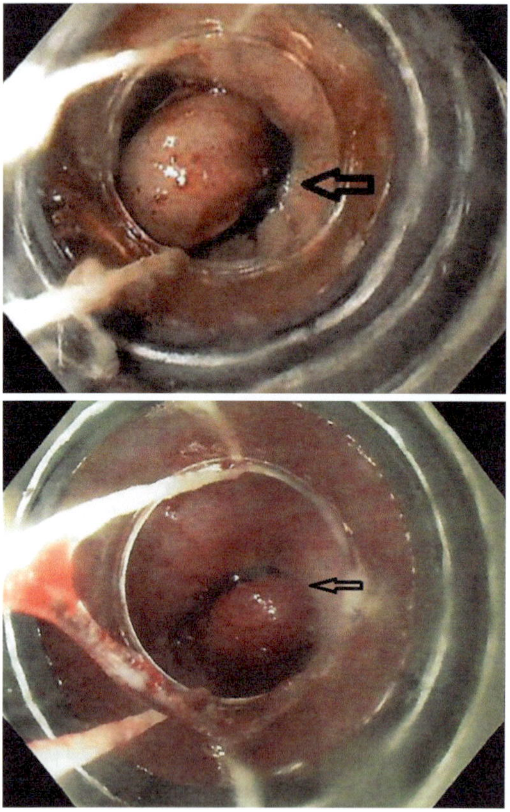

FIGURE 5.3 AND 5.4 Varix post band ligation therapy visualized through an endoscope. Shown are two images of esophageal varices post band ligation therapy visualized through the banding apparatus via endoscopy. Note black rubber band at neck of each varix (arrow) post procedure

therapy should be repeated at intervals until varices are no longer visible, thereby reducing the risk of bleeding [14].

Portal hypertension can be associated with changes affecting the lining of the stomach known as portal hypertensive gastropathy (see Fig. 5.5) and can also result in the formation of gastric varices (see Fig. 5.6). Gastric varices are not typically treated with band ligation, but these may require transjugular intrahepatic portosystemic stent shunt (TIPS) placement if beta-blockers are not tolerated or bleeding recurs [9]. TIPS implantation is performed by an interventional radiologist under x-ray guidance. A device that creates a conduit between the portal vein with elevated pressures and the outflow through the hepatic vein is inserted within the liver to establish communication between these two circulations. By creating an alternative pathway for blood flow, a reduction in the pressure in the portal circulation occurs [28]. One other treatment for gastric varices is the use of cyanoacrylate "glue" for obliterating the gastric varices [9]. This is not uniformly performed at most centers and does carry

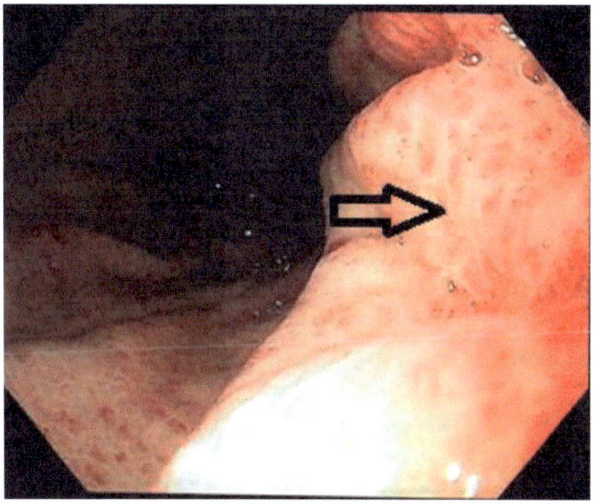

FIGURE 5.5 Portal hypertensive gastropathy. The image demonstrates the lining of the stomach with a mosaic like appearance that resembles snakeskin, consistent with changes of portal hypertensive gastropathy

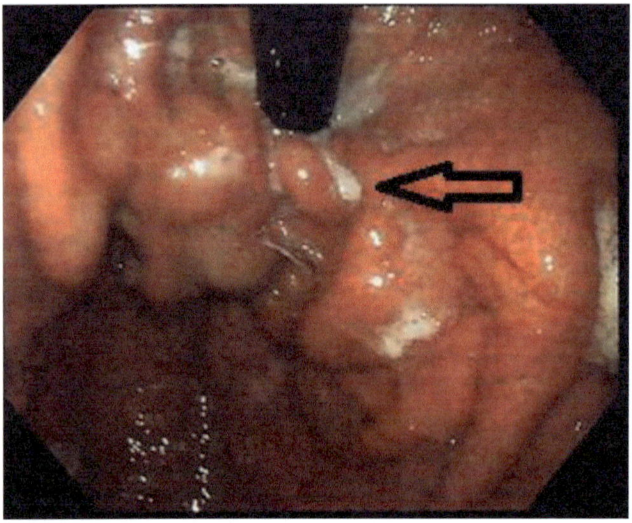

FIGURE 5.6 Gastric varices with portal hypertensive gastropathy. Shown are gastric varices at the gastric fundus visualized on retroflexion of the endoscope (arrow)

other risks as well. Surgical shunts to decompress the portal system were performed more commonly in the past but are infrequent now due to the success of the TIPS procedure. One other alternative for treating gastric varices is balloon-occluded retrograde transvenous obliteration (BRTO), performed by interventional radiologists, where the presence of spontaneous connections between the high-pressure portal system and the systemic venous system can be used as a conduit to access the portal system and the varices closed off by use of coils or special glues or sclerosing agents [15, 16].

Management of Variceal Bleed

Active bleeding can present with hematemesis (vomiting blood) or passing melena (black stool containing altered blood). This situation can be life-threatening with a high mortality rate and requires emergent hospitalization and care as detailed. When active bleeding from varices occurs, volume resuscitation and airway protection (sometimes requiring placement of an endotracheal tube and use of a ventilator) are needed. Patients should undergo emergency endoscopy and intravenous infusions of medications such as octreotide or vasopressin (that reduce portal blood flow) as required to control the bleeding, as well as treatment with antibiotics to prevent complications of SBP and sepsis that often accompany the bleeding episode. Admission to an intensive care unit is needed for support and monitoring. If bleeding is uncontrolled, then TIPS may be considered as an option for emergently reducing the bleeding from varices.

Ascites

Portal hypertension may result in the retention of salt and water and fluid shifts outside the vascular space, clinically seen as swelling initially in the lower extremities (edema) and by abdominal distension with ascites. Ascites and edema can be treated with sodium restriction and diuretics, a class of medications which cause increased loss of salt and water in the urine. The initial diuretic used is often the aldosterone antagonist spironolactone [24]. Some male patients may experience discomfort from breast enlargement (gynecomastia) due to the hormonal action of spironolactone, and alternative diuretics may be needed. If the ascites and edema are not adequately reduced, the addition of a second-loop diuretic (e.g., furosemide) can be considered [4]. Sodium restriction and sufficient protein intake (1.2–1.5 g/kg/day) have also been recommended as an adjunct to treatment [18]. Careful monitoring of renal function and electrolytes on initiation and during dose adjustments is required to prevent electrolyte imbalance and deterioration of kidney function.

Deterioration in kidney function can also occur independently of diuretic use in patients with advanced liver disease with significant portal hypertension. This progressive deterioration in kidney function, in the absence of any identifiable triggers, is referred to as hepatorenal syndrome (HRS).

Treatments available for HRS include stopping medications that can contribute to deteriorating kidney function, volume expansion of the plasma with albumin given intravenously, treatment with analogues of vasopressin, placement of TIPS, and dialysis [11, 31]. Despite treatment initiation, mortality remains high in patients with HRS, and prognosis without transplantation is poor [2].

Treatment of Resistant Ascites

If medications are not effective at improving the ascites or in patients that are unable to tolerate diuretics, the ascitic fluid may require direct drainage (abdominal paracentesis). This is a simple bedside procedure performed most often in an outpatient setting, where a needle or catheter is inserted into the peritoneal cavity to directly remove the excess fluid. In cases where medications to control ascites are ineffective or not tolerated due to side effects and where regular paracentesis becomes necessary due to rapid fluid re-accumulation, placement of a TIPS by nonsurgical methods can be considered to reduce portal pressures and ascites [22, 23], alongside evaluation for liver transplantation. Patients with a history of uncontrolled hepatic encephalopathy (see below) as well as cardiac and pulmonary disease may need careful consideration prior to TIPS insertion due to a risk of deterioration after the shunt is placed [12].

Spontaneous Bacterial Peritonitis

Patients with advanced liver disease with ascites have a reduced resistance to infection and have an increased frequency of passage of bacteria across the gut wall (increased bacterial translocation). Ascites can become infected and result in the development of spontaneous bacterial peritonitis (SBP). SBP can present with abdominal pain or with features of overwhelming infection that include bacterial or toxin spread in the circulation causing sepsis associated with fever, rapid heart rate, low blood pressure, and sometimes reduced oxygen saturation. Diagnosis is by analysis of ascites fluid by paracentesis, demonstrating most often an increase in white blood cells in the ascites above 250 granulocytes per microliter or less commonly by a positive microbial culture [21]. Treatment is with antibiotics, intravenous infusion of albumin to preserve kidney function, and supportive care. Diuretics are held during treatment of SBP. Once SBP occurs in an individual, patients may be advised to continue an oral antibiotic on a daily or weekly basis to prevent further episodes from occurring.

Sepsis

Patients with advanced liver cirrhosis are also at a higher risk of other bacterial infections, and these are one of the main causes of hospitalization. [13] This reflects an impaired immune system occurring due to advanced liver disease. SBP and urinary tract infections are the most frequent infections, followed by pneumonia, skin and soft tissue infections, and bacteremia [13]. Gram-negative bacteria from intestinal origin can play a role in a considerable proportion of patients, yet gram-positive bacteria are a frequent cause in hospitalized patients. Atypical and even fungal pathogens need to be considered in patients not responding to treatment. Early diagnosis and prompt initiation of appropriate antibiotics or antifungal treatment are essential [7].

Hepatic Encephalopathy

One of the primary roles of a functioning liver is that it metabolizes potentially toxic substances in the body to make them harmless. When the liver does not fully function due to scarring and bypass of the normal circulation through the liver or with severe inflammation and impairment of normal metabolism, toxins can build up in the blood stream. The accumulation of certain toxins and chemicals such as ammonia can precipitate a condition known as hepatic encephalopathy with resulting brain dysfunction and altered mental status. The finding of a raised serum ammonia level can support the diagnosis of hepatic encephalopathy. There are a range of symptoms of hepatic encephalopathy, beginning with an altered sleep-wake cycle and progressing to altered mentation and daytime drowsiness. This can evolve further to difficulty in responding to the patient's surroundings and eventually to a full-blown coma state. The earliest stages of hepatic encephalopathy, now called subclinical or minimal hepatic encephalopathy, can be detected by standardized neuropsychiatric tests [30]. Overt hepatic encephalopathy is detected by altered mentation and the pres-

TABLE 5.3 Stages of hepatic encephalopathy

	Stage	**State of consciousness**	**Clinical symptoms**	**Exam findings**
Covert	0	Normal	None	Normal examination
	1	Mild lack of awareness	Altered sleep pattern	Altered mental acuity on testing, impaired addition or subtraction, mild asterixis or tremor
Overt	2	Lethargy or apathy	Mild disorientation, forgetful, inappropriate behavior	Obvious asterixis, slurred speech, altered mental acuity
	3	Somnolent but arousable	Drowsy, severe disorientation	Somnolent, altered mentation
	4	Comatose	Not arousable	Not arousable

This table based on the West Haven criteria of Hepatic Encephalopathy. It demonstrates the various stages of encephalopathy and the progression from covert to overt symptoms (Adapted from Bajaj et al. [5]).

ence of a flapping tremor (asterixis) (see Table 5.3 for stages of hepatic encephalopathy).

Management of hepatic encephalopathy focuses initially on identifying and treating a precipitating cause. Hepatic encephalopathy is made worse by medications that are sedating, variceal bleeding, infection or constipation, the latter due to buildup of toxins and ammonia generated by the gut bacteria, or by kidney dysfunction. Medications to reduce ammonia levels and improve clearance of nitrogenous waste products absorbed in the gut can also be used. In mild cases, a simple laxative such as lactulose can reduce the production of ammonia by converting the energy source of gut bacteria to lactulose instead of protein [3, 20], as well as by its effect to increase bowel movements due to an osmotic diarrhea (the undigested sugar reduces fluid absorption by the gut). In severely impaired patients that cannot take lactulose by mouth, encouraging bowel movement with enema treatments (tap water or with lactulose) can help clear the buildup of nitrogenous waste products. Non-absorbed antibiotics such as rifaximin or neomycin are another treatment option for hepatic encephalopathy that are thought to eliminate ammonia-producing colonic bacteria [6]. Due to its increased safety profile, rifaximin is used more often than neomycin which has been associated with kidney dysfunction and hearing loss in some patients. Often a combination of treatments, lactulose and a non-absorbed antibiotic, is used. In severe hepatic encephalopathy resulting in a comatose state, supportive measures including mechanical ventilation can be required. After an episode of hepatic encephalopathy, secondary prophylaxis to prevent future episodes is recommended using lactulose and occasionally rifaximin [30].

Malignancy

Occasionally symptoms such as jaundice, abdominal pain, variceal bleeding, and bleeding into abdominal space (hemoperitoneum) can suggest a more sinister underlying cause such as the development of hepatocellular carcinoma (primary liver cancer). Hepatocellular carcinoma (HCC) is a recognized complication of liver cirrhosis and can occur even in patients with compensated disease, though most often with advancing portal hypertension. Although the risk for developing liver cancer in Wilson disease appears to be lower than for other etiologies of cirrhosis [19], expert opinion recommends screening on a 6-month basis with ultrasonography imaging and analysis of the tumor marker alpha-fetoprotein. Occasionally alternative dynamic imaging such as computerized tomography (CT) or magnetic resonance imaging (MRI) may be performed for further characterization if results of the ultrasound examination are inconclusive or suspicious for an abnormal finding. The purpose of screening and surveillance is to detect a liver tumor at a time when it can be treated effectively, by surgery or by ablation or with liver transplantation. HCC can be asymptomatic or present with symptoms that resemble decompensated liver disease. Tumor infiltration of the liver with HCC can result in worsening jaundice. Abdominal pain can be a feature resulting from enlargement of the tumor mass causing pressure on the liver capsule. Complications of portal hypertension (variceal bleeding, ascites, and encephalopathy) can worsen in the presence of an HCC due to occlusion of the hepatic vein which drains the liver. Obstruction can occur either by direct tumor infiltration or due to blood clot formation from a prothrombotic state. Hepatocellular carcinomas are hypervascular, and spontaneous rupture is a complication that is seen in 3–15% of cases [29]. In patients with a coagulopathy due to poor liver synthetic function from cirrhosis and tumor invasion, this complication can cause hemoperitoneum, often with peritonitis and hemodynamic instability resulting in a poor prognosis.

Another less common liver tumor is cholangiocarcinoma that arises from bile duct cells. These can also present with a deep jaundice which is cholestatic in nature due to the tumor location causing obstruction of the biliary drainage system. Methods of relieving the obstruction include stenting of the biliary tree by endoscopic retrograde cholangiopancreatography (ERCP) or with external drainage systems placed using percutaneous transhepatic cholangiography (PTC). These tumors can be very aggressive, but if found at an early stage and localized to the liver, surgical resection may be possible.

Acute Liver Failure

In some instances, disease progression in undiagnosed Wilson disease follows a more rapid course resulting in liver failure. Acute liver failure can also occur in those who were previously treated but who have discontinued their medications. Symptoms from acute liver failure include a rapid onset of jaundice, an altered level of consciousness due to encephalopathy, and sometimes stomach discomfort from abdominal swelling with ascites. A telltale sign for WD is anemia from rupturing red blood cells and the release of their contents, a process known as hemolysis. Untreated liver failure in Wilson disease carries an almost 95% mortality. Liver transplantation must be considered and a referral made emergently to a transplant center. A discussion of liver transplant for Wilson disease follows in a separate chapter.

Bibliography

1. Aigner E, Theurl I, Haufe H, Seifert M, Hohla F, Scharinger L, Stickel F, Mourlane F, Weiss G, Datz C. Copper availability contributes to iron pertubations in human nonalcoholic fatty liver disease. Gastroenterology. 2008;135:680–8.
2. Alessandria C, Ozdogan O, Guevara M, Restuccia T, Jiménez W, Arroyo V, Rodés J, Ginès P. MELD score and clinical type predict prognosis in hepatorenal syndrome: relevance to liver transplantation. Hepatology. 2005;41(6):1282.
3. Als-Nielsen B, Gluud LL, Gluud C. Non-absorbable disaccharides for hepatic enephalopathy: systemic review of randomised trials. BMJ. 2004;328(7447):1046.
4. Angeli P, Fasolato S, Mazza E, Okolicsanyi L, Maresio G, Velo E, Galioto A, Salinas F, D'Aquino M, Sticca A, Gatta A. Combined versus sequential diuretic treatment of ascites in non-azotaemic patients with cirrhosis: results of an open randomised clinical trial. Gut. 2010;59(1):98–104.
5. Bajaj JS, Frederick RT, Bass NM, Ghabril M, Coyne K, Margolis MK, Santoro M, Coakley DF, Mokhtarani M, Jurek M, Scharschmidt BF. Overt hepatic encephalopathy: development of a novel clinician reported outcome tool and electronic caregiver diary. Metab Brain Dis. 2016;31:1081–93.

6. Bass NM, Mullen KD, Sanyal A, Poordad F, Neff G, Leevy CB, Sigal S, et al. Rifaximin treatment in hepatic encephalopathy. N Engl J Med. 2010;362(12):1071–81.
7. Fagiouli S, Colli A, Bruno R, Burra P, Craxì A, Gaeta GB, Grossi P, Mondelli MU, Puoti M, Sagnelli E, Stefani S, Toniutto P. Management of infections in cirrhotic patients: report of a consensus conference. Dig Liver Dis. 2014;46(3):204–12.
8. Ferenci P, Caca K, Loudianos G, Mieli-Vergani G, Tanner S, Sternlieb I, Schilsky M, Cox D, Berr F. Diagnosis and phenotypic classification of Wilson disease. Liver Int. 2003;23:139–42.
9. Garcia-Pagan JC, Barrufet M, et al. Management of gastric varices. Clin Gastroenterol Hepatol. 2014;12(6):919–28.
10. Garcia-Tsao G, Abraldes JG, Berzigotti A, Bosch J. Portal hypertensive bleeding in cirrhosis: risk stratification, diagnosis and management: 2016 practice guidance by the American Assoication for the study of liver diseases. Hepatology. 2017;65:310–35.
11. Gines P, Guevara M, Arroyo V, Rodés J. Hepatorenal syndrome. Lancet. 2003;362:1819.
12. Gollon JL, Gollan TJ. Wilson disease in 1998: genetic, daignostic and therapeutic aspects. J Hepatol. 1998;28:28–36.
13. Jalan R, Fernandez J, Wiest R, Schnabl B, Moreau R, Angeli P, Stadlbauer V, Gustot T, Bernardi M, Canton R, Albillos A, Lammert F, Wilmer A, Mookerjee R, Vila J, Garcia-Martinez R, Wendon J, Such J, Cordoba J, Sanyal A, Garcia-Tsao G, Arroyo V, Burroughs A, Ginès P. Bacterial infections in cirrhosis: a position statement based on EASL special conference. J Hepatol. 2013;60(6):1310–24.
14. Jutabha R, Jensen DM, Martin P, Savides T, Han SH, Gornbein J. Randomized study comparing banding and propranolol to prevent initial variceal hemorrhage in cirrhotics with high risk esophageal varices. Gastroenterology. 2005;128(4):870–81.
15. Kim SK, Lee KA, Sauk S, Korenblat K. Comparison of transjugular intrahepatic portosystemic shunt with covered stent and balloon-occluded retrograde transvenous obliteration in managing isolated gastric varices. Korean J Radiol. 2017;18(2):345–54.
16. Lee SJ, Kim SU, Kim MD, Kim YH, Kim GM, Park SI, Won JY, Lee DY, Lee KH. Comparison of treatment outcomes between ballooon-occluded retrograde transvenous obliteration and transjugular intrahepatic portosystemic shunt for gastric variceal bleeding hemostasis. J Gastroenterol Hepatol. 2017;32(8):1487–94.

17. Merle U, Schaefer M, Ferenci P, Stremmel W. Clinical presentation, diagnosis and long term outcome of Wilson's disease: a cohort study. Gut. 2007;56:115–20.
18. Peng S, Plank LD, McCall JL, Gillanders LK, McIlroy K, Gane EJ. Body composition, muscle function, and energy expenditure in patients with liver cirrhosis: a comprehensive study. Am J Clin Nutr. 2007;85(5):1257–66.
19. Pfeiffenberger J, Mogler C, Gotthardt DN, Schulze-Bergkamen H, Litwin T, Reuner U, Hefter H, Huster D, Schemmer P, Członkowska A, Schirmacher P, Stremmel W, Cassiman D, Weiss KH. Hepatobiliary malignancies in Wilson disease. Liver Int. 2015;35(5):1257–66.
20. Rahimi RS, Singal AG, Cuthbert JA, Rockey DC. Lactulose vs polyethylene glycol 3350 – electrolyte solution for treatment of overt hepatic encephalopathy: the HELP randomized clinical trial. JAMA Intern Med. 2014;174(11):1727–33.
21. Rimola A, García-Tsao G, Navasa M, Piddock LJ, Planas R, Bernard B, Inadomi JM. Diagnosis, treatment and prophylaxis of spontaneous bacterial peritonitis: a consensus document. *International Ascites Club*. J Hepatol. 2000;32(1):142–53.
22. Rossle M, Ochs A, Gülberg V, Siegerstetter V, Holl J, Deibert P, Olschewski M, Reiser M, Gerbes AL. A comparison of paracentesis and transjugular intrahepatic portosystemic shunting in patients with ascites. N Engl J Med. 2000;342(23):1701–7.
23. Salerno F, Merli M, Riggio O, Cazzaniga M, Valeriano V, Pozzi M, Nicolini A, Salvatori F. Randomized controlled study of TIPS versus paracentesis plus albumin in cirrhosis with severe ascites. Hepatology. 2004;40(3):629–35.
24. Santos J, Planas R, Pardo A, Durández R, Cabré E, Morillas RM, Granada ML, Jiménez JA, Quintero E, Gassull MA. Spironolactone alone or in combination with frusemide in the treatment of moderate ascites in nonazotemic cirrhosis. A randomized comparative study of efficacy and safety. J Hepatol. 2003;39(2):187–92.
25. Stattermayer AF, Traussnigg S, Dienes HP, Aigner E, Stauber R, Lackner K, Hofer H, Stift J, Wrba F, Stadlmayr A, Datz C, Strasser M, Maieron A, Trauner M, Ferenci P. Hepatic steatosis in Wilson disease – role of copper and PNPLA3 mutations. J Hepatol. 2015;63:156–63.
26. Stemmel W, Meyerrose KW, Niederau C, Hefter H, Kreuzpaintner G, Strohmeyer G. Wilson's disease: clinical presentation, treatment and survival. Ann Intern Med. 1991;115:720–6.

27. Turnes J, Garcia-Pagan JC, Abraldes JG, Hernandez-Guerra M, Dell'Era A, Bosch J. Pharmacological reduction of portal pressure and long-term risk of first variceal bleeding in patients with cirrhosis. Am J Gastroenterol. 2006;101(3):506–12.
28. Unger LW, Berlakovich GA, Trauner M, Reiberger T. Management of portal hypertension before and after liver transplantation. Liver Transpl. 2018;24(1):112–21.
29. Vergara V, Muratone A, Bouzari H. Spontaneous rupture of hepatocellular carcinoma: surgical resection and long-term survival. Eur J Surg Oncol. 2000;26:770–2.
30. Vilstrup H, Amodio P, Bajaj J, Cordoba J, Ferenci P, Mullen KD, et al. Hepatic encephalopathy in chronic liver disease: 2014 practice guideline by the American Association for the Study of Liver Diseases and the European Association for the Study of the liver. Hepatology. 2014;60(2):715–35.
31. Wadei HM, Mai ML, Ahsan N, Gonwa TA. Hepatorenal syndrome: pathophysiology and management. Clin J Am Soc Nephrol. 2006;1(5):1066–79.

Chapter 6
Treatment of Neurological Symptoms in Wilson Disease

Ana Vives-Rodriguez, Daphne Robakis, and Nigel S. Bamford

Introduction

Neurological symptoms are extremely common in Wilson disease (WD), occurring as the initial manifestation of WD in 40–70% of cases [1–6]. Patients that present initially with neurological symptoms usually have a later onset than patients with initial liver manifestations, exhibiting symptoms in their 20s [1, 6–9].

Current de-coppering therapy provides in most cases only partial improvement of the neurological aspects of WD, and, in 10–15% of cases, there can be an initial worsening of neurological symptoms after starting therapy [6]. For these reasons, the use of medications to treat residual neurological symptoms often improves patients' quality of life. However, few studies assess the efficacy of these medications. This chapter aims to

A. Vives-Rodriguez (✉) · D. Robakis
Department of Neurology, Yale University, New Haven, CT, USA
e-mail: ana.vives-rodriguez@yale.edu

N. S. Bamford
Department of Neurology, Yale University, New Haven, CT, USA

Department of Pediatrics, Yale University, New Haven, CT, USA

Department of Cellular and Molecular Physiology, Yale University, New Haven, CT, USA

M. L. Schilsky (ed.), *Management of Wilson Disease*, Clinical Gastroenterology, https://doi.org/10.1007/978-3-319-91527-2_6

TABLE 6.1 Summary of symptomatic therapeutic options for neurological manifestations of Wilson disease

Neurological manifestations	Clinical features	Treatment Options
Action tremor	Tremor present with manual activities or with arms outstretched against gravity (kinetic and postural tremor)	Propranolol 20–240 mg daily, divided into two or three doses Primidone 25–750 mg daily, divided into two or three doses
Dystonia	Focal dystonia (involving one body part)	Botulinum toxin injections every 12 weeks. Dose will depend on location and severity
	Multifocal or generalized dystonia	Trihexyphenidyl Starting dose: 1–2 mg daily Usual effective dose: 8–30 mg daily divided into two or three doses Baclofen Starting dose 10 mg daily Usual effective dose: 60–120 mg daily divided into two or three doses
Parkinsonism	Masked face, rigidity, bradykinesia, resting tremor	Levodopa 300–1200 mg per day divided into three doses
Ataxia	Dysarthria, incoordination, dysmetria, broad-based gait	Physical therapy, speech therapy, home safety evaluation
Sialorrhea	Hypersalivation	Botulinum toxin injections every 12 weeks

review the most common neurological manifestations in WD and the therapeutic options currently available (Table 6.1).

Neurological Manifestations of WD

For unclear reasons, copper accumulation in the brain centers in the basal ganglia and brainstem structures which modulate movements [10, 11]. Therefore, many of the neurological manifestations of WD are movement disorders such as tremor, dysarthria, parkinsonism, dystonia, or gait impairment. Other neurological manifestations that have been described less frequently include epilepsy, neuropathy, and headaches [1, 12, 13].

The diagnosis of WD in a patient with initial neurologic manifestations requires a high clinical suspicion. At first, patients may seek medical evaluation for non-specific symptoms such as learning difficulties, anxiety, or tremor. Therefore, physicians who suspect WD should order a comprehensive neurological examination. Laboratory investigations often include a ceruloplasmin level that is the major copper-carrying protein in the blood. Additional studies often include serum and urine copper levels, liver and renal function studies, and a complete blood count. With high clinical suspicion, an ophthalmological evaluation is performed, where a slit-lamp examination can detect copper deposition in the iris, known as Kayser-Fleischer rings. Brain imaging studies (discussed below) should be considered.

A patient with a suspected or confirmed diagnosis of WD should be referred to a neurologist for evaluation. The most common neurological manifestations of WD and treatment options are summarized in Table 6.1.

Tremor

Tremor is a predominant neurologic feature, presenting in approximately half (39–83%) of WD patients [3, 6, 13, 14]. Some authors describe tremor as the most frequent neurological manifestation of WD [9]. It can involve the head, arms, or legs. Tremor can be present at rest, when the patient is not performing any activities, or with action. At first, it often appears during manual activities such as writing, getting dressed, or pouring liquids (called kinetic tremor) or when the patient is holding the arms outstretched against gravity (called postural tremor) [6, 9]. As the disease progresses, the tremor may adopt other characteristics such as a "wing-beating" tremor. This is a high-amplitude tremor present with arms abducted and flexed at the elbows. Tremor can also accompany other neurological manifestations such as dystonia, cerebellar ataxia, and parkinsonism, which will be discussed in the following sections.

Symptomatic treatment can be tried if the tremor is bothersome to the patient or if it is interfering with fine motor activities or other activities of daily living. Only case series and case reports have addressed the effect that standard anti-tremor medications have on WD tremor [15–17]. Therefore, these medications are often used as off-label indications, based on the characteristics of the tremor.

Medications for Action Tremor

If tremor demonstrates a more postural and kinetic quality, medications classically used for this type of tremor might be tried. Propranolol is usually the first line of treatment for action tremor given its low incidence of side effects and low risk of interaction with other medications. The dose that has been typically used ranges from 20 to 240 mg daily, and it is usually divided into two or three doses per day. Its most common side effects are bradycardia and hypotension. Therefore, an initial low dose and slow titration are recommended [18, 19].

Primidone is another medication frequently used for other types of action tremor. Nevertheless, it is extensively metabolized by the liver, therefore its use in the WD population should be considered with caution, especially in patients with impaired liver function. Other medications that have some evidence for the treatment of tremor are benzodiazepines, gabapentin and topiramate. However, the benefit in WD tremor is unknown.

Dystonia

Dystonia has been reported in a wide range of patients with WD (18–65%) [3, 13, 14] and has been described as the most disabling and refractory neurological feature [1, 6, 9, 20]. Dystonia is a neurological disorder characterized by involuntary sustained muscle contractions that cause twisting, repetitive movements, and abnormal postures [21]. It can involve any body part such as the face, neck, trunk, and limbs. Sustained muscle contraction involving the face and jaw causing jaw opening or forced fixed smile is known as risus sardonicus. These abnormal muscle contractions may interfere with eating, performing manual activities, standing, and walking. In some cases, dystonia is accompanied by a dystonic tremor.

Dystonic tremor is characterized by a postural or kinetic tremor that occurs in a body region affected by dystonia [22, 23]. Some clues that can aid this diagnosis are abnormal posturing in the hands with arms outstretched such as asymmetric flexion or extension of the wrists or fingers, improvement of the tremor in certain positions (hands pronated vs supinated), or the presence of abnormal postures in adjacent body parts such as the neck.

Treatment Options for Dystonia

Medications that have been commonly used for the treatment of dystonia are botulinum toxin, anticholinergics, and baclofen. The treatment of choice is going to depend on the distribution of the dystonia.

Botulinum Toxin Injections

Botulinum toxin is the first line of treatment for focal dystonia (dystonia affecting one isolated body part) because of its high efficacy and low rate of side effects. Botulinum toxin is directly injected into the affected muscle to produce paralysis, thus avoiding any systemic side effects. After the injection of the toxin, an effect is expected within 3 days, with a peak effect at 2 weeks, and is completely reversible. Patients may require periodic injections every 3 months [24, 25]. Side effects can be related to the injection, such as bruising or pain, or they can be associated to the toxin effect, such as excessive muscle weakness, dysphagia (if the neck is injected), double vision (if the face is injected), or flu-like symptoms that can appear a few days after the injections are performed [25].

Botulinum toxin can also be directly injected to the salivary glands to reduce excessive salivation or drooling which is a common complaint of patients with WD.

Oral Medications

Oral medications are recommended in patients with dystonia or dystonic tremor that involves multiple regions of the body. Botulinum toxin is generally not recommended in these cases due to the high dose of toxin and number of injections required and the increased likelihood of systemic side effects. The most commonly used oral drugs for dystonia are anticholinergics and baclofen [26].

Trihexyphenidyl (Artane) is the only anticholinergic with sufficient evidence supporting its use in dystonia [27, 28]. Trihexyphenidyl should be started at a low dose of 1–2 mg daily and weekly titrated to a usual effective dose of 8–30 mg per day, divided into two or three doses per day [17]. It is generally well tolerated in younger patients even at high doses, but adults are more sensitive to side effects [29]. Common side effects are dry mouth, constipation, blurred vision, slowness in thinking, and urinary retention.

Baclofen is effective for the treatment of dystonia due to its muscle relaxant effects. It should be started at a low dose of 10 mg daily and up-titrated slowly to an average dose of 60–120 mg daily [26, 27]. Its main side effects are drowsiness, nausea, and dizziness. The dose should be tapered slowly when discontinuing treatment. Combined therapy with anticholinergics can be considered.

Parkinsonism

Parkinsonism is a clinical syndrome characterized by the combination of rigidity, resting tremor, bradykinesia, and postural instability [24]. Parkinsonism is present in about half (38–62%) of WD cases. Masked face, bradykinesia, postural imbalance, and cogwheel rigidity are the most common parkinsonian features documented [6]. A rest tremor in the hands or legs can be seen in patients with WD, but it is rare [6], and when present, it is generally asymmetric [9].

The medication that is most commonly used for parkinsonian features is levodopa. It is prescribed as a combination of levodopa and carbidopa (Sinemet). Carbidopa inhibits the peripheral metabolism of levodopa so is added to increase efficacy and improve tolerability. In some countries, the available formulation consists of benserazide rather than carbidopa.

There are no reports that systematically assess the response of parkinsonian features seen in WD to levodopa or dopamine agonists. Nevertheless, in patients with significant parkinsonian signs, a trial of levodopa can be offered. A small dose of carbidopa/levodopa (25 mg/100 mg) three times a day can be initiated and slowly increased, at weekly intervals, to 1200 mg of levodopa per day to determine responsiveness [30]. The patient should be monitored for side effects, mainly nausea, orthostatic hypotension, hallucinations, and impulse control disorders.

Cerebellar Ataxia

Cerebellar ataxia as a feature of WD has been documented in roughly one third (28–51%) of the patients [4, 6, 13]. The cerebellum is a brain structure that modifies the quality of movement to make them harmonious and precise. Ataxia is the medical term used to describe incoordination of fine motor activities that leads to clumsiness with under- or overshooting of the limbs as they attempt to reach a precise target. Tremor can also be a feature of cerebellar ataxia. This tremor is known as intention tremor. It is absent at rest and present with action, with worsening of its amplitude when approaching a visual target, as when performing finger-to-nose maneuvers. Ataxia can also involve the trunk (titubation) and lead to significant postural instability and increased fall risk. Dysarthria, or slurred speech, is commonly encountered in patients with WD, but its neurological origin appears to be multifactorial and arises secondary to cerebellar ataxia, dystonia, and/or parkinsonism [10, 22].

At present, no pharmacological therapy has proven effective for the treatment of ataxia. Physiotherapy-based interventions, such as balance, postural control, gait training, and the use of compensatory orthotics and aids, may be offered to patients.

Dysphagia

Patients with WD frequently have trouble swallowing; such difficulties are reported in half of cases with neurological manifestations. Dysphagia may be due to impairment of chewing, swallowing, and esophageal motility which are related to incoordination, slowness, and weakness of deglutition muscles [9, 31].

Dysphagia can lead to aspiration pneumonia, weight loss, and malnutrition [32]. Therefore, the physician should inquire about this symptom at every visit and obtain a swallow function evaluation as soon as such difficulties are suspected. Monitoring of the patient's nutritional status by weight, calorie counts, and laboratory-based measurements are also recommended.

Neurological Manifestations in Children

While WD patients most frequently present with symptoms during adolescence and young adulthood, symptom onset can occur in a broad age range that includes toddlers and young children [7, 33–35].

Hepatic liver disease is the most common presentation of WD in children and is most frequently suspected by detecting hepatosplenomegaly on examination or by abnormal liver function tests incidentally found during routine blood studies [36]. However, there are several reports of children and young adolescents with neurological manifestations at disease onset. Tremor, dystonia, dysarthria, and deterioration of school performance are the features most frequently described [13, 36, 37]. Symptoms can be subtle and non-specific at first; thus a high index of suspicion is required to make a timely diagnosis. Younger at-risk patients may be identified early by obtaining a positive family history of the disease.

Clinical Scales Used for Neurological Evaluation of WD

Neurologists rely on clinical rating scales as tools to quantify changes in the neurological examination over time. This is important in Wilson disease for the objective assessment of response to chelating therapy and symptomatic treatment. In the last decade, two scales have been published and validated for the assessment of neurological manifestations of WD: the Unified Wilson Disease Rating Scale (UWDRS) and the Global Assessment Scale (GAS) for WD [38, 39]. The UWDRS includes a comprehensive neurological assessment and a questionnaire to assess activities of daily living and functionality. The GAS, in addition to the neurological assessment, includes liver disease and psychiatric and cognitive symptoms evaluation. Both scales are validated tools for the clinical assessment of WD patients in clinical and research settings [40].

Neuroimaging in WD

Current practice guidelines recommend radiologic imaging of the brain, preferably by magnetic resonance imaging (MRI), in all patients with neurologic WD [41, 42]. Almost all patients with neurological manifestations of the disease demonstrate abnormalities on brain MRI, with hyperintense lesions in the basal ganglia, thalamus, and pons in T2-weighted and FLAIR sequences being most frequently reported [2, 43–45]. Hyperintense and hypointense lesions in the basal ganglia in T1-weighted images have also been described [43, 46]. It is important to add that roughly half (42–70%) of patients with only hepatic manifestations and 20% of asymptomatic patients can also have MRI abnormalities [44, 45]. Findings described on imaging are not specific for WD. Therefore, additional testing, such as laboratory screening, a liver biopsy, or an ophthalmological examination, maybe needed to confirm the diagnosis. The utility of performing routine MRI after starting treatment is unclear and is not performed in clinical practice.

Conclusion

Neurological manifestations of WD can involve multiple domains of the central nervous system with movement disorders being most frequently encountered. Despite the removal of excess copper by chelating agents, residual neurological symptoms often persist in WD patients. Treating residual neurological signs and symptoms in WD is challenging but can significantly improve quality of life. Little has been written about specific treatments for the neurological manifestations of this condition, and further research in this area is needed.

Bibliography

1. Brewer GJ, Yuzbasiyan-Gurkan V. Wilson disease. Medicine (Baltimore). 1992;71(3):139–64.
2. Starosta-Rubinstein S, Young AB, Kluin K, Hill G, Aisen AM, Gabrielsen T, et al. Clinical assessment of 31 patients with Wilson disease. Correlations with structural changes on magnetic resonance imaging. Arch Neurol. 1987;44(4):365–70.

3. Dastur DK, Manghani DK, Wadia NH. Wilson disease in India. I. Geographic, genetic, and clinical aspects in 16 families. Neurology. 1968;18(1 Pt 1):21–31.
4. Taly AB, Meenakshi-Sundaram S, Sinha S, Swamy HS, Arunodaya GR. Wilson disease: description of 282 patients evaluated over 3 decades. Medicine (Baltimore). 2007;86(2):112–21.
5. Huang CC, Chu NS. Wilson disease: clinical analysis of 71 cases and comparison with previous Chinese series. J Formos Med Assoc Taiwan Yi Zhi. 1992;91(5):502–7.
6. Lorincz MT. Neurologic Wilson disease. Ann N Y Acad Sci. 2010;1184:173–87.
7. Merle U, Schaefer M, Ferenci P, Stremmel W. Clinical presentation, diagnosis and long-term outcome of Wilson disease: a cohort study. Gut. 2007;56(1):115–20.
8. Oder W, Grimm G, Kollegger H, Ferenci P, Schneider B, Deecke L. Neurological and neuropsychiatric spectrum of Wilson disease: a prospective study of 45 cases. J Neurol. 1991;238(5):281–7.
9. Członkowska A, Litwin T, Chabik G. Wilson disease: neurologic features. Handb Clin Neurol. 2017;142:101–19.
10. Nazer H, Brismar J, al-Kawi MZ, Gunasekaran TS, Jorulf KH. Magnetic resonance imaging of the brain in Wilson disease. Neuroradiology. 1993;35(2):130–3.
11. Algin O, Taskapilioglu O, Hakyemez B, Ocakoglu G, Yurtogullari S, Erer S, et al. Structural and neurochemical evaluation of the brain and pons in patients with Wilson disease. Jpn J Radiol. 2010;28(9):663–71.
12. Zimbrean PC, Schilsky ML. Psychiatric aspects of Wilson disease: a review. Gen Hosp Psychiatry. 2014;36(1):53–62.
13. Machado A, Chien HF, Deguti MM, Cançado E, Azevedo RS, Scaff M, et al. Neurological manifestations in Wilson disease: report of 119 cases. Mov Disord Off J Mov Disord Soc. 2006;21(12):2192–6.
14. Stremmel W, Meyerrose KW, Niederau C, Hefter H, Kreuzpaintner G, Strohmeyer G. Wilson disease: clinical presentation, treatment, and survival. Ann Intern Med. 1991;115(9):720–6.
15. Brewer GJ, Fink JK, Hedera P. Diagnosis and treatment of Wilson disease. Semin Neurol. 1999;19(3):261–70.
16. Hölscher S, Leinweber B, Hefter H, Reuner U, Günther P, Weiss KH, et al. Evaluation of the symptomatic treatment of residual neurological symptoms in Wilson disease. Eur Neurol. 2010;64(2):83–7.

17. Litwin T, Dušek P, Członkowska A. Symptomatic treatment of neurologic symptoms in Wilson disease. Handb Clin Neurol. 2017;142:211–23.
18. Louis ED. Diagnosis and management of tremor. Contin Minneap Minn. 2016;22(4 Movement Disorders):1143–58.
19. Ondo W. Essential tremor: what we can learn from current pharmacotherapy. Tremor Hyperkinetic Mov N Y N. 2016;6:356.
20. Svetel M, Kozić D, Stefanova E, Semnic R, Dragasevic N, Kostic VS. Dystonia in Wilson disease. Mov Disord Off J Mov Disord Soc. 2001;16(4):719–23.
21. Marsden CD, editor. Movement disorders: neurology 2: Buttwerworth-Heinemann Oxford, UK; 2013. 394 p.
22. Deuschl G. Dystonic tremor. Rev Neurol (Paris). 2003;159(10 Pt 1):900–5.
23. Fasano A, Bove F, Lang AE. The treatment of dystonic tremor: a systematic review. J Neurol Neurosurg Psychiatry. 2014;85(7):759–69.
24. Fahn S, Jankovic J, Hallett M. Principles and practice of movement disorders, vol. 3330: Elsevier Health Sciences Saunders Elsevier Philadelphia, USA; 2011.
25. Pellizzari R, Rossetto O, Schiavo G, Montecucco C. Tetanus and botulinum neurotoxins: mechanism of action and therapeutic uses. Philos Trans R Soc Lond B Biol Sci. 1999;354(1381):259–68.
26. Dressler D, Altenmueller E, Bhidayasiri R, Bohlega S, Chana P, Chung TM, et al. Strategies for treatment of dystonia. J Neural Transm Vienna Austria 1996. 2016;123(3):251–8.
27. Thenganatt MA, Jankovic J. Treatment of dystonia. Neurother J Am Soc Exp Neurother. 2014;11(1):139–52.
28. Maltese M, Martella G, Madeo G, Fagiolo I, Tassone A, Ponterio G, et al. Anticholinergic drugs rescue synaptic plasticity in DYT1 dystonia: role of M1 muscarinic receptors. Mov Disord Off J Mov Disord Soc. 2014;29(13):1655–65.
29. Fahn S. High dosage anticholinergic therapy in dystonia. Neurology. 1983;33(10):1255–61.
30. McFarland NR. Diagnostic approach to atypical Parkinsonian syndromes. Contin Minneap Minn. 2016;22(4 Movement Disorders):1117–42.
31. da Silva-Júnior FP, Carrasco AE a B, da Silva Mendes AM, Lopes AJT, Nobre E Souza MA, de Bruin VMS. Swallowing dysfunction in Wilson disease: a scintigraphic study. Neurogastroenterol Motil Off J Eur Gastrointest Motil Soc. 2008;20(4):285–90.

32. Członkowska A, Tarnacka B, Litwin T, Gajda J, Rodo M. Wilson disease-cause of mortality in 164 patients during 1992–2003 observation period. J Neurol. 2005;252(6):698–703.
33. Wilson DC, Phillips MJ, Cox DW, Roberts EA. Severe hepatic Wilson disease in preschool-aged children. J Pediatr. 2000;137(5):719–22.
34. Iorio R, D'Ambrosi M, Mazzarella G, Varrella F, Vecchione R, Vegnente A. Early occurrence of hypertransaminasemia in a 13-month-old child with Wilson disease. J Pediatr Gastroenterol Nutr. 2003;36(5):637–8.
35. Tissières P, Chevret L, Debray D, Devictor D. Fulminant Wilson disease in children: appraisal of a critical diagnosis. Pediatr Crit Care Med J Soc Crit Care Med World Fed Pediatr Intensive Crit Care Soc. 2003;4(3):338–43.
36. Roberts EA, Socha P. Wilson disease in children. Handb Clin Neurol. 2017;142:141–56.
37. Noureen N, Rana MT. Neurological Wilson disease in children: a three years experience from Multan. JPMA J Pak Med Assoc. 2011;61(8):743–8.
38. Członkowska A, Tarnacka B, Möller JC, Leinweber B, Bandmann O, Woimant F, et al. Unified Wilson disease rating scale – a proposal for the neurological scoring of Wilson disease patients. Neurol Neurochir Pol. 2007;41(1):1–12.
39. Leinweber B, Möller JC, Scherag A, Reuner U, Günther P, Lang CJG, et al. Evaluation of the Unified Wilson Disease Rating Scale (UWDRS) in German patients with treated Wilson disease. Mov Disord Off J Mov Disord Soc. 2008;23(1):54–62.
40. Volpert HM, Pfeiffenberger J, Gröner JB, Stremmel W, Gotthardt DN, Schäfer M, et al. Comparative assessment of clinical rating scales in Wilson disease. BMC Neurol. 2017;17(1):140.
41. Roberts EA, Schilsky ML, American Association for Study of Liver Diseases (AASLD). Diagnosis and treatment of Wilson disease: an update. Hepatol Baltim Md. 2008;47(6):2089–111.
42. European Association for Study of Liver. EASL clinical practice guidelines: Wilson disease. J Hepatol. 2012;56(3):671–85.
43. Ranjan A, Kalita J, Kumar S, Bhoi SK, Misra UK. A study of MRI changes in Wilson disease and its correlation with clinical features and outcome. Clin Neurol Neurosurg. 2015;138:31–6.
44. King AD, Walshe JM, Kendall BE, Chinn RJ, Paley MN, Wilkinson ID, et al. Cranial MR imaging in Wilson disease. AJR Am J Roentgenol. 1996;167(6):1579–84.

45. Litwin T, Dzieżyc K, Poniatowska R, Członkowska A. Effect of liver transplantation on brain magnetic resonance imaging pathology in Wilson disease: a case report. Neurol Neurochir Pol. 2013;47(4):393–7.
46. Kim TJ, Kim IO, Kim WS, Cheon JE, Moon SG, Kwon JW, et al. MR imaging of the brain in Wilson disease of childhood: findings before and after treatment with clinical correlation. Am J Neuroradiol. 2006;27(6):1373–8.

Chapter 7
Psychiatric Aspects of Wilson Disease

Sahil Munjal and Paula C. Zimbrean

Introduction

The psychiatric manifestations of Wilson disease (WD) have been reported since the original paper by Samuel Alexander Kinnier Wilson (1878–1937) was published in 1912 [1]. In his report, Wilson describes psychiatric symptoms in 8 of 12 cases and "schizophrenia-like psychosis" in 2 of the cases. Other reports describe a wide spectrum of psychiatric disorders, including cognitive impairment [2–4], dementia [5], mental retardation, anxiety [6], "schizophrenia-like states" [7], and behavior abnormalities and personality disorders [8], suicidality [6, 9], and obsessive–compulsive disorder [10]. In children and adolescents, reports of psychiatric symptoms with Wilson disease are rare and include psychosis [11] and non-specific behavioral difficulties [12, 13].

S. Munjal · P. C. Zimbrean (✉)
Department of Psychiatry, Yale University School of Medicine, New Haven, CT, USA
e-mail: Sahil.Munjal@yale.edu; Paula.Zimbrean@yale.edu

M. L. Schilsky (ed.), *Management of Wilson Disease*, Clinical Gastroenterology, https://doi.org/10.1007/978-3-319-91527-2_7

The estimated lifetime prevalence of psychiatric symptoms in WD patients varies widely, between 30 and 100% among symptomatic patients [8].The reason for this variability includes reports by clinicians without mental health training, use of ill-defined terminologies, lack of prospective evaluation, assessment during remission phase, and lack of information regarding diagnostic criteria [14].

Due to the variety of psychiatric symptoms described in patients with WD, the illness has been called "a great masquerader" [15]. In this chapter, we are going to discuss relevant aspects of the clinical evaluation of psychiatric symptoms in WD (depressive disorders, bipolar and related disorders, anxiety disorders, psychosis, personality issues, other relevant behavior abnormalities such as nonadherence), prevalence of psychiatric symptoms, significance of psychiatric symptoms, and treatment considerations.

Evaluation of Psychiatric Symptoms in WD

Psychiatric symptoms in WD had been typically believed to be present along with neurological symptoms, and patients were labeled as having neuropsychiatric disturbances. More recently, however, it became apparent that neurologic and psychiatric symptoms do not always present concurrently. Psychiatric evaluations traditionally rely primarily on the patient interview, on the patient's report of internal experiences, and on mental status evaluation. When neurological problems are present, they can impact the psychiatric evaluation in multiple ways: any significant speech impairment can affect communication and reduces the information that can be obtained from the patient. Memory difficulties, when present, render history taken unreliable. Neurological symptoms may be confused with psychiatric symptoms (e.g., bradykinesia being mistaken for psychomotor retardation, a sign of depression). Medications used for neurological symptoms in WD may have side effects that present like psychiatric symptoms (e.g., benzodiazepines and lethargy).

When the liver function is significantly impaired, the presence of hepatic encephalopathy may preclude a proper psychiatric evaluation and delay an accurate diagnosis. Hepatic encephalopathy (HE) represents a broad continuum of neuropsychiatric abnormalities, from subtly altered mental status to deep coma, seen in patients with liver dysfunction. As a neuropsychiatric disorder, HE affects consciousness, personality, behavior, emotion and affect, memory, and cognition [16, 17]. These symptoms may mimic almost all of the major psychiatric syndromes: delirium, dementia, confusion, anxiety, depression, mania, and psychosis or personality disorder [18, 19] rendering the diagnosis of underlying psychiatric disorder more difficult.

In order to mitigate these difficulties in accurately diagnosing psychiatric problems in WD patients, two major tools must be considered: extensive collateral information from family members, friends, and previous providers and the use of structured psychiatric assessments. Patient's family, previous medical providers, and hospital records can be extremely helpful in obtaining a good history of psychiatric symptoms and the relationship with coexisting neurological and active liver disease. In addition to obtaining a detailed history of the psychiatric and medical symptoms, collateral information my produce helpful information about the patient's adjustment to having WD. The mental health clinician must pay attention to cognitive distortions such as denial of illness and to health related behaviors (e.g., adherence with treatment or lack of their off). It is not uncommon to see patients who have suffered with psychiatric symptoms for many years to almost embrace the WD diagnosis when finally found and attribute all prior difficulties to the disease, which may not always be accurate. For instance, somebody with antisocial personality disorder may readily accept WD as the main cause for their poor judgment and impulsivity and disregard the fact that WD alone does not explain fully their personality traits. In addition to detailed collateral information, the use of structured instruments can help in assessing psychiatric problems in patients with WD. At this time, there are no psychiatric scales that have been fully validated in this population. Below we discuss some instruments which have been studied extensively in patients with chronic medical illness and have been used in WD. Most of these instruments have been used extensively in primary care settings and can be administered by nonmental health clinicians, such as primary care providers or nurses. If the patients screen positive, they should be referred to a facility where they will be appropriately diagnosed, treated with evidence-based psychiatric treatment with adequate follow-up [20].

Patient health questionnaire 9 (PHQ-9) is a 9-item self-report questionnaire that can help to detect the presence of depression and supplement a thorough psychiatric and mental health interview. It scores the 9 *Diagnostic and Statistical Manual of Mental Disorders, Fifth Edition* (DSM-5) criteria for depression on a scale of 0 (not at all) to 3 (nearly every day). It is a public resource that is easily available online without any cost. PHQ-9 has shown excellent test–retest reliability in screening for depression, and normative data on the instrument's use are available in various clinical populations [21].

In one study, a PHQ-9 score of ≥10 had 88% sensitivity and specificity for detecting depression, with scores of 5, 10, 15, and 20 indicating mild, moderate, moderately severe, and severe depression, respectively [22]. In addition to its use as a screening tool, PHQ-9 is a good measure of depression treatment outcomes [23]. It has been used to assess depression in WD population [24].

Generalized Anxiety Disorder 7-item scale (GAD 7) is a brief, self-administered questionnaire for screening and measuring severity of GAD [25]. It asks patients to rate seven items that represent problems with general anxiety and scores each item on a scale of 0 (not at all) to 3 (nearly every day). Sensitivity and specificity are 89% and 82%, respectively [26]. It performs well for detecting and monitoring not only GAD but also panic disorder, social anxiety disorder, and posttraumatic stress disorder [27].

Mood Disorder Questionnaire (MDQ) is another brief, self-report questionnaire that is available on the internet. It is designed to identify and monitor patients who are likely to meet diagnostic criteria for bipolar disorder [28, 29]. The first question on the MDQ asks if the patient has experienced any of 13 common mood and behavior symptoms. The second question asks if these symptoms have ever occurred at the same time, and the third asks the degree to which the patient finds the symptoms to be problematic. The remaining two questions provide additional clinical information, because they address family history of manic–depressive illness or bipolar disorder and whether a diagnosis of either disorder has been made. It has a specificity of >97% which means that it will effectively screen out just about all true negatives [28].

Several other rating scales are readily available which are brief, useful, and easy to incorporate into clinical practice which may be helpful for not only screening of psychiatric problems, but, also for monitoring the trajectory of the treatment. Few others include Columbia Suicide Severity Rating Scale (C-SSRS) for evaluation of suicidality, HAM-D Hamilton Depression Rating Scale and Beck Depression Inventory (BDI) for depression, Adult ADHD Self-Report Scale (ASRS) for ADHD, Montreal Cognitive Assessment (MOCA), Mini-Mental Status Evaluation (MMSE), etc.

Prevalence and Significance of Psychiatric Symptoms in WD

Some authorities have speculated that psychiatric symptoms indicate a more severe or advanced disease, may be related to irreversible brain damage secondary to copper toxicity, or are secondary to alternative metabolic influences produced by the malfunction of the liver such as hyperammonemia associated with hepatic encephalopathy [6]. Many patients with WD will have psychiatric symptoms develop after diagnosis and initiation of treatment or following lapses in therapy [30]. WD is characterized by chronic course and need of treatments, impairment of functional outcomes, and high frequency of psychiatric symptoms. Some reports showed a link between presence of bipolar disorders diagnosis, cerebral damage, and low quality of life (QOL) [31]. Recognition of the relationship of the psychiatric symptoms to WD can help with administration of appropriate therapy aimed at both the psychiatric issues and underlying WD. Therefore, knowledge of the psychiatric aspects of WD is essential for psychiatrists and other medical professionals practicing in a general hospital setting.

It has been reported that the median time for initial presentation to diagnosis for patients with psychiatric symptoms alone was 2.4 years (S.D. =2.9), much higher than for neurologic WD (1.5 years) or hepatic WD (0.5 years) [9, 32].

The causes for delay in diagnosis are varied in literature [30, 33]. Walshe and Yealland [33] attributed these to underestimation and lack of awareness among treating physicians and laboratory errors in estimation of copper and ceruloplasmin levels. They emphasized that KF rings should be evaluated by an experienced ophthalmologist, using a slit lamp. Further, it is important to recognize that KF rings may not be present when illness manifests with non-neuropsychiatric features.

There is not much literature, and further investigation is indicated to better understand the manifestation of Wilson's heterozygous disease, with special emphasis on psychiatric symptoms.

Cognitive Impairment

Memory change is one of the most common impairments, but other cognitive changes have been reported, including dementia in untreated cases [34], impairment in executive function, working memory, and abstract reasoning [35]. Several clinical accounts have described cases of WD which showed cognitive abnormalities leading to functional impairment, corresponding to clinical features that resemble a dementia syndrome [1, 5, 36].

Patients showing neurological motor symptoms usually also present with, from the outset, changes in behavior or cognitive decline [33]. This decline appears in approximately 25% of the patients [37]. Depending on the test used and whether the patients present with more hepatic or neurological symptoms, this figure can reach up to 40% [33, 38]. Patients suffering from WD show a significantly poorer performance on global cognitive tests such as the Mini-Mental State Examination [38] and the Mattis Dementia Rating Scale [39] compared to healthy voluntary participants. Memory deficits have been described by several authors [3, 39, 40]. These authors have found that patients suffering from WD show lower capacity to both learn words and recall them across all stages of the Rey Auditory-Verbal Learning Test (RAVLT).

Although initially considered irreversible, the association of Wilson disease with irreversible cognitive decline is no longer the rule in the context of effective medical therapy for the disorder [32].

Depression

Prevalence of depression and in patients with WD varies between 4% and 47% [41]. Depression seems to be correlated with alterations of serotoninergic transmission in the thalamus–hypothalamus and midbrain–pons region, in particular with low density of the presynaptic serotonin transporter (SERT) [42].

In psychiatry, we make distinction between MDD and other types of depression, such as dysthymia and adjustment disorders. When symptoms are considered to be exclusive to a medical condition, we call it "depression secondary to another medical condition." The essential feature of depressive disorder due to another medical condition is a prominent and persistent period of depressed mood or markedly diminished interest or pleasure in all, or almost all, activities that predominates in the clinical picture (Criterion A) and that is thought to be related to the direct physiological effects of another medical condition (Criterion B). In determining whether the mood disturbance is due to a general medical condition, the clinician must first establish the presence of a general medical condition. Further, the clinician must establish that the mood disturbance is etiologically related to the general medical condition through a physiological mechanism. There are a couple of considerations to keep in mind. One consideration is the presence of a temporal association between the onset, exacerbation, or remission of the general medical condition and that of the mood disturbance. A second consideration is the presence of features that are atypical of primary mood disorders (e.g., atypical age at onset, sudden onset, or absence of family history).

Adjustment disorders define the presence of psychiatric symptoms such as depression or anxiety in reaction to a clear identified stressor. According to DSM-5, the reaction must occur within 3 months of the onset of the stressor(s). These symptoms or behaviors are clinically significant, as evidenced by one or both of the following: marked distress that is out of proportion to the severity or intensity of the stressor and significant impairment in social, occupational, or other important areas of functioning. The clinician must take into account the external context and the cultural factors that might influence symptom severity and presentation. In order to be diagnosed as adjustment disorder, the stress-related disturbance does not meet the criteria for another mental disorder and is not merely an exacerbation of a preexisting mental disorder. Once the stressor or its consequences have terminated, the symptoms do not persist for more than an additional 6 months. Adjustment disorders can present with depressed mood, anxiety, mixed depressed mood and anxiety, disturbance of conduct, mixed disturbance of emotions and conduct, and unspecified. It is important to note that in many cases depression has been described in the beginning of clinical manifestations of WD, before the disease cost disability, financial burden, or relationship problems. Therefore in many cases, depression cannot be exclusively attributed to an adjustment to coping with the chronic disease.

The most common and most likely treated type of depression is major depressive disorder (MDD). In order to diagnose an episode of MDD, five or more symptoms from the following must be present nearly every day during same 2-week period: depressed mood most of the day, nearly daily, diminished interest or pleasure, excessive or inappropriate guilt or feelings of worthlessness, fatigue or loss of energy, difficulty concentrating, significant weight loss (5% of body weight in 1 month) or decrease or increase in appetite, psychomotor agitation, insomnia/hypersomnia and/or thoughts of death, or suicidal thoughts or behaviors [43].

The essential feature of persistent depressive disorder (dysthymia) is a depressed mood that occurs for most of the day, for more days than not, for at least 2 years or at least 1 year for children and adolescents [43]. Only two cohort studies have described specific types of depressive disorders in WD patients: Shanmugiah (2008) found that 4% of patients with WD had major depressive disorder while 2% met the diagnostic criteria for dysthymic disorder [44]. More recently, Carta et al. found that 47.8% of patient with WD met criteria for major depressive disorder [45].

Bipolar Disorders and Bipolar Spectrum

Bipolar presentations can vary from a full manic episode (which includes abnormally and persistently elevated, expansive, or irritable mood, persistently increased goal-directed activity or energy, inflated self-esteem or grandiosity, decreased need for sleep, more talkative or pressure to keep talking, flight of ideas or subjective racing thoughts, distractibility, increase in goal-directed activity activities with high potential for bad consequences and last for at least a week) to various degrees of mood instability or impulsivity. Prevalence of bipolar disorder in patients with WD varies between 18% and 39% [41]. In addition to formally diagnosed bipolar disorders, patients with WD may present with various degree of mood instability that may not meet criteria for mania or hypomania but may significantly impact the quality of life [9, 45].

It is also important to know that WD patients may present at various points in their lives with behavioral changes that do not meet criteria for specific psychiatric disease [46]: irritability (prevalence 15–25%) [47, 48], impaired social judgment or disinhibition [9, 48], apathy [48], "belligerence" [9], or "incongruent behavior" [47]. Personality changes are described in up to 57% of patients with WD [8, 47].

Differentiating psychiatric symptoms in WD from an underlying primary psychiatric disorder is extremely challenging. Features that point toward psychiatric symptoms being secondary to WD are coexistence between psychiatric symptoms and neurological or liver disease, abrupt onset of psychiatric symptoms, psychiatric symptoms not meeting the criteria for common DSM-5 syndromes, and evidence of laboratory or brain imaging abnormalities. Distinguishing between primary psychiatric disease and psychiatric symptoms secondary to WD may guide the length of treatment as we will discuss below.

Psychosis

Psychosis has been described at various points in the course of WD and has included frank delusions and/or thought disorder or disorganized thinking [49–53]. In a cohort of 71 Chinese patients with WD, 11.3% had been diagnosed with schizophrenia [54]. Cases have been reported of patients carrying the diagnosis of schizophrenia for years, prior to being diagnosed with WD. Psychosis may result in refusal of WD treatment, and this vicious circle can lead to deterioration of patient's neurological state. It is not fully clear whether the resolution of psychosis in these patients is caused by antipsychotic or WD medication.

Suicidality

There is no formal data about the rate of suicide in patients with WD. For psychiatric illness, the estimated lifetime suicide rate varies from about 15% for major depressive disorder [55] to 6% for schizophrenia [55] and 4% for alcoholism [55]. Any mental health evaluation must include a thorough safety assessment. If the patient has any suicidal ideations, the clinician must assess access to means, active intent, lethality of means, method, onset, frequency, intensity, duration, precipitants, and plans. The presence of psychotic symptoms, command hallucinations, severe anxiety, and alcohol or substance use, history and seriousness of previous attempts, and family history of or recent exposure to suicide must be also evaluated. If patient is deemed to be an immediate risk, arrangements must be made for urgent psychiatric care and constant observation. This may include transfer to a psychiatric emergency room and psychiatric unit and psychiatric commitment; however provided that safety is ensured, the least restrictive setting is preferred. Acute treatment should consist of establishing therapeutic rapport, targeting modifiable risk factors, involving friends and family, and establishing safety plan (versus a safety contract) and discharge plan if hospitalized [55].

Disease Detection and Pathogenesis

Establishing a diagnosis of WD is crucial since early detection and treatment may prevent disease progression and even reverse damage in some patients. About 40% of all patients with WD first present with liver abnormalities, 40% with neurological abnormalities, and 20% with psychiatric abnormalities [56]. 10% to 20% of patients present with psychiatric disorders 1–5 years before the diagnosis of WD, and one-third of these patients receive psychiatric treatment, including hospitalization [8].

There are not enough studies to guide us in determining the extent of evaluation for WD that should be implemented in the general psychiatric population for patients at their first presentation [57]. Recent guidelines recommend that Wilson disease should be ruled out in any patient with hepatic impairment, irrespective of severity, in combination with any neurological or neuropsychiatric manifestation [58].

Screening for WD in psychiatric patients via ceruloplasmin levels has been attempted [59]; however, results were not promising due to the lack of sensitivity of the testing [60].

A recent study was done to evaluate the relevance of serum copper (Cu) and ceruloplasmin (Cp) measures in hospitalized patients with psychiatric disorders and to identify possible mutations in the ATP7B gene in patients with abnormal biological copper profile. Results of ceruloplasmin and/or serum Cu concentrations below the normal limits are common in patients with psychiatric disorders and nonrelevant and/or informative for the WD diagnosis [61].

Screening tests for all suspected patients are covered in other chapters on disease diagnosis but should include slit-lamp examination for KF ring by an experienced ophthalmologist, abdominal ultrasound for architectural changes in the liver, and the use of serum copper, ceruloplasmin, and 24-h urinary copper from a reliable laboratory [62]. Kayser–Fleischer rings are an important diagnostic sign; unfortunately it is not present in all WD patients, not even when neurological disease is noticeable [63, 64].

The mechanism of psychiatric symptoms in Wilson disease is not clear. Because symptoms can occur at the start of the illness, they are not fully explained by the psychosocial impact of a medical condition. Initially it was thought that basal ganglia abnormalities led to various psychiatric symptoms through dopamine dysregulation. More recent studies have explored the role of copper and other microelements in schizophrenia and bipolar illness [65, 66].

Treatment of Psychiatric Symptoms in WD

Although it is well recognized that WD often presents with psychiatric problems, little is known about the treatment or the prognosis of these clinical manifestations. Two treatment approaches to psychiatric symptoms in WD patients have been described [32]:

1. Primary treatment of Wilson disease directed at removal of pathological copper deposition (chelation therapy or treatment with zinc) alone leads to an improvement in psychiatric symptoms [67, 68]. Up to one-third of patients with psychiatric symptoms will improve with de-coppering treatment alone [46]. Modai et al. reported on d-penicillamine efficacy in acute psychotic disorders [68].
2. Psychotropic medication or psychotherapy is used to address specific psychiatric presentations independent of medical therapy for WD. Trials of various psychotropic medications have been reported, including lithium, haloperidol, tricyclic antidepressants, benzodiazepines, quetiapine, risperidone, and clozapine, as well as trials of ECT [41, 52, 69, 70]. It should be noted that high incidences of neurological side effects caused by psychotropic medications have been reported in patients with WD [71].

Typical or atypical antipsychotics have been used to good clinical effect with the overall warning that WD patients are very sensitive to neuroleptics and prone to develop extrapyramidal symptoms [41]. There is evidence supporting the practice of selecting antipsychotics that are less likely to cause extrapyramidal symptoms (such as quetiapine) and titrating the dosage slowly [32]. Clozapine [69], quetiapine [70], and olanzapine [72] have been used effectively to treat symptoms in patients with WD with psychiatric manifestations. But severe extrapyramidal syndrome had been reported with the use of neuroleptics [72].

Since lenticular (source of dopamine) degeneration is the hallmark of this disorder, dopamine is already depleted in the affected regions. With the addition of atypical antipsychotics (which blocks nigrostriatal dopamine), already depleted basal ganglia are further deprived of dopamine. This could also explain the sensitivity of the patients to atypical antipsychotics. Also, patients with WD are more vulnerable to agranulocytosis due to hypersplenism and/or d-penicillamine. It has been reported that there is an increased risk of neutropenia and agranulocytosis with concomitant use of d-penicillamine and neuroleptics [73]. Clozapine, sometimes used in WD patients [69], might not be a suitable option in such patients as it can enhance the risk of agranulocytosis.

Bipolar disorder has been treated with a combination of lithium and olanzapine, which has led to a gradual mood stabilization and successful recovery [74]. Lithium is a preferred agent as a mood stabilizer, considering its renal excretion and many of these patients have significant hepatic dysfunction. It also stimulates granulocyte production and might be a much safer option over clozapine in certain patients [75]. However, it should be prescribed with caution as it may exaggerate the tremor.

ECT in control of acute psychosis of WD has also been reported, especially in patients who have extrapyramidal symptoms along with psychosis as neuropsychiatric symptoms of WD [76].

There have been cases when penicillamine or zinc sulfate was reported as useful for psychiatric symptoms [77], without any employment of neuroleptic medications [78].

Patients with WD may have active medical problems requiring prompt management that psychiatric units often are not equipped to provide. Close collaboration with the medical team is essential in the long-term management of these patients. Often a psychiatrist in a consultative role follows patients with WD when they are hospitalized on a medical unit [32].

Colocated models of care have been reported to improve the quality of life of patients with liver [79] and neurological disease [80]. This model, which implies the presence of mental health professionals in the medical clinic, needs to be considered for WD because of the high prevalence of psychiatric symptoms. WD Centers for Excellence provide physicians who are well trained in the diagnosis and treatment of WD, physician training and research regarding WD, broad services needed by WD patients and their families, multidisciplinary treatment, and technical support required by patients [81]. Psychoeducation and/or referral to support organizations, such as the Wilson Disease Association, can ease the burden on caregivers.

There are no data to guide the duration of treatment with psychotropics in WD, since there have been no systematic studies of the correlation of biological markers with psychiatric symptoms in the disorder. Close ongoing observation is advocated to identify when the psychiatric symptoms resolve and the disease markers are normalized. At that time, attempts should be made to discontinue the psychotropic medications to reduce short- and long-term side effects.

The results showing the impact of liver transplantation upon psychiatric symptoms in WD are mixed. There have been cases of psychiatric improvement after orthotopic liver transplantation (OLT) [82]. Studies also have shown neuropsychiatric problems may worsen after liver transplantation [83] or leaving them unchanged [84, 85]. At this time, liver transplantation is not recommended for treatment of neuropsychiatric symptoms in WD in the absence of liver impairment.

Many studies have demonstrated motor and cognitive improvement after initiating clinical treatment for WD. This observation led to WD being categorized as a reversible dementia, both after clinical treatment [5, 36] or after hepatic transplant [86]. The association of WD with irreversible cognitive decline is no longer the rule in the context of effective medical therapy for the disorder [41].

Summary

Psychiatric manifestations represent a significant part of the clinical presentation of WD. They can present at any point in the course of the illness, including in the absence of hepatic or neurologic involvement, leading to delays or misdiagnosis of WD. They should be carefully evaluated from the patient interview, using collateral information from family members, friends, and previous providers, and the use of structured psychiatric instruments. Establishing a diagnosis of WD is crucial since early detection and treatment may prevent disease progression and even reverse damage in some patients.

Good outcomes can be expected with specific therapies for WD, adherence to medicaments, and clinical monitoring. Along with therapy directed at the prevention of accumulation and the removal of copper, treatment of psychiatric symptoms in Wilson disease may require psychotropic medications. Selecting psychotropics that are less likely to cause extrapyramidal symptoms and titrating the dosage slowly are the preferred approaches. The aim of care should be full recovery, since patients may maintain remission for years after psychotropic medications have been discontinued.

Bibliography

1. Wilson SAK. Progressive lenticular degeneration: a familial nervous disease associated with cirrhosis of the liver. Brain. 1912;34(4):295–507.
2. Bornstein RA, McLean DR, Ho K. Neuropsychological and electrophysiological examination of a patient with Wilson disease. Int J Neurosci. 1985;26(3–4):239–47.
3. Seniow J, Bak T, Gajda J, Poniatowska R, Czlonkowska A. Cognitive functioning in neurologically symptomatic and asymptomatic forms of Wilson disease. Mov Disord. 2002;17(5):1077–83.
4. Portala K, Levander S, Westermark K, Ekselius L, von Knorring L. Pattern of neuropsychological deficits in patients with treated Wilson disease. Eur Arch Psychiatry Clin Neurosci. 2001;251(6):262–8.
5. Rosselli M, Lorenzana P, Rosselli A, Vergara I. Wilson disease, a reversible dementia: case report. J Clin Exp Neuropsychol. 1987;9(4):399–406.
6. Rathbun JK. Neuropsychological aspects of Wilson disease. Int J Neurosci. 1996;85(3–4):221–9.
7. Saint-Laurent M. Schizophrenia and Wilson disease. Can J Psychiatr. 1992;37(5):358–60.
8. Akil M, Brewer GJ. Psychiatric and behavioral abnormalities in Wilson disease. Adv Neurol. 1995;65:171–8.
9. Oder W, Grimm G, Kollegger H, Ferenci P, Schneider B, Deecke L. Neurological and neuropsychiatric spectrum of Wilson disease: a prospective study of 45 cases. J Neurol. 1991;238(5):281–7.

10. Kumawat BL, Sharma CM, Tripathi G, Ralot T, Dixit S. Wilson disease presenting as isolated obsessive-compulsive disorder. Indian J Med Sci. 2007;61(11):607–10.
11. McDonald LV, Lake CR. Psychosis in an adolescent patient with Wilson disease: effects of chelation therapy. Psychosom Med. 1995;57(2):202–4.
12. Carr A, McDonnell DJ. Wilson disease in an adolescent displaying an adjustment reaction to a series of life stressors: a case study. J Child Psychol Psychiatry. 1986;27(5):697–700.
13. Crumley FE. Pitfalls of diagnosis in the early stages of Wilson disease. J Am Acad Child Adolesc Psychiatry. 1990;29(3):470–1.
14. Srinivas K, Sinha S, Taly AB, Prashanth LK, Arunodaya GR, Janardhana Reddy YC, et al. Dominant psychiatric manifestations in Wilson disease: a diagnostic and therapeutic challenge! J Neurol Sci. 2008;266(1–2):104–8.
15. Soltanzadeh A, Soltanzadeh P, Nafissi S, Ghorbani A, Sikaroodi H, Lotfi J. Wilson disease: a great masquerader. Eur Neurol. 2007;57(2):80–5.
16. Ferenci P, Lockwood A, Mullen K, Tarter R, Weissenborn K, Blei AT. Hepatic encephalopathy--definition, nomenclature, diagnosis, and quantification: final report of the working party at the 11th world congresses of gastroenterology, Vienna, 1998. Hepatology. 2002;35(3):716–21.
17. Frederick RT. Current concepts in the pathophysiology and management of hepatic encephalopathy. Gastroenterol Hepatol (N Y). 2011;7(4):222–33.
18. Rosenberg R, Renvillard SG, Hjerrild S. Organic delirious states and other psychiatric disorders: lessons for the hepatologists. Metab Brain Dis. 2013;28(2):235–8.
19. Groeneweg M, Quero JC, De Bruijn I, Hartmann IJ, Essink-bot ML, Hop WC, et al. Subclinical hepatic encephalopathy impairs daily functioning. Hepatology. 1998;28(1):45–9.
20. Siu AL, Bibbins-Domingo K, Grossman DC, Baumann LC, Davidson KW, Ebell M, et al. Screening for depression in adults: US preventive services task force recommendation statement. JAMA. 2016;315(4):380–7.
21. Patient Health Questionnaire. Available from: http://www.agencymeddirectors.wa.gov/files/AssessmentTools/14- PHQ-9%20 overview.pdf
22. Kroenke K, Spitzer RL, Williams JB. The PHQ-9: validity of a brief depression severity measure. J Gen Intern Med. 2001;16(9):606–13.

23. Lowe B, Unutzer J, Callahan CM, Perkins AJ, Kroenke K. Monitoring depression treatment outcomes with the patient health questionnaire-9. Med Care. 2004;42(12):1194–201.
24. Schaefer M, Gotthardt DN, Ganion N, Wohnsland S, Seessle J, Stremmel W, et al. Wilson disease: health-related quality of life and risk for depression. Clin Res Hepatol Gastroenterol. 2016;40(3):349–56.
25. Spitzer RL, Kroenke K, Williams JB, Lowe B. A brief measure for assessing generalized anxiety disorder: the GAD-7. Arch Intern Med. 2006;166(10):1092–7.
26. Lowe B, Decker O, Muller S, Brahler E, Schellberg D, Herzog W, et al. Validation and standardization of the Generalized Anxiety Disorder Screener (GAD-7) in the general population. Med Care. 2008;46(3):266–74.
27. Kroenke K, Spitzer RL, Williams JB, Monahan PO, Lowe B. Anxiety disorders in primary care: prevalence, impairment, comorbidity, and detection. Ann Intern Med. 2007;146(5):317–25.
28. Ketter TA. Strategies for monitoring outcomes in patients with bipolar disorder. Prim Care Companion J Clin Psychiatry. 2010;12(Suppl 1):10–6.
29. Texas Uo. Mood disorder questionnaire. Available from: http://www.dbsalliance.org/pdfs/MDQ.pdf
30. Prashanth LK, Taly AB, Sinha S, Arunodaya GR, Swamy HS. Wilson disease: diagnostic errors and clinical implications. J Neurol Neurosurg Psychiatry. 2004;75(6):907–9.
31. Carta MG, Sorbello O, Moro MF, Bhat KM, Demelia E, Serra A, et al. Bipolar disorders and Wilson disease. BMC Psychiatry. 2012;12:52.
32. Zimbrean PC, Schilsky ML. The spectrum of psychiatric symptoms in Wilson disease: treatment and prognostic considerations. Am J Psychiatry. 2015;172(11):1068–72.
33. Walshe JM, Yealland M. Wilson disease: the problem of delayed diagnosis. J Neurol Neurosurg Psychiatry. 1992;55(8):692–6.
34. Frota NAF, Caramelli P, Barbosa ER. Cognitive impairment in Wilson disease. Dement Neuropsychol. 2009;3(1):16–21.
35. Wenisch E, De Tassigny A, Trocello JM, Beretti J, Girardot-Tinant N, Woimant F. Cognitive profile in Wilson disease: a case series of 31 patients. Rev Neurol (Paris). 2013;169(12):944–9.
36. Riley D, Wiznitzer M, Schwartz S, Zinn AB. A 13-year-old boy with cognitive impairment, retinoblastoma, and Wilson disease. Neurology. 2001;57(1):141–3.

37. Lauterbach EC, Cummings JL, Duffy J, Coffey CE, Kaufer D, Lovell M, et al. Neuropsychiatric correlates and treatment of lenticulostriatal diseases: a review of the literature and overview of research opportunities in Huntington's, Wilson's, and Fahr's diseases. A report of the ANPA Committee on Research. American Neuropsychiatric Association. J Neuropsychiatry Clin Neurosci. 1998;10(3):249–66.
38. Sinha S, Christopher R, Arunodaya GR, Prashanth LK, Gopinath G, Swamy HS, et al. Is low serum tocopherol in Wilson disease a significant symptom? J Neurol Sci. 2005;228(2):121–3.
39. Medalia A, Isaacs-Glaberman K, Scheinberg IH. Neuropsychological impairment in Wilson disease. Arch Neurol. 1988;45(5):502–4.
40. Isaacs-Glaberman K, Medalia A, Scheinberg IH. Verbal recall and recognition abilities in patients with Wilson disease. Cortex. 1989;25(3):353–61.
41. Zimbrean PC, Schilsky ML. Psychiatric aspects of Wilson disease: a review. Gen Hosp Psychiatry. 2014;36(1):53–62.
42. Loudianos G, Gitlin JD. Wilson disease. Semin Liver Dis. 2000;20(3):353–64.
43. Depressive Disorders. Diagnostic and statistical manual of mental disorders: DSM Library: Arlington, VA: American Psychiatric Association. 2013.
44. Shanmugiah A, Sinha S, Taly AB, Prashanth LK, Tomar M, Arunodaya GR, et al. Psychiatric manifestations in Wilson disease: a cross-sectional analysis. J Neuropsychiatr Clin Neurosci. 2008;20(1):81–5.
45. Carta MG, Farina GC, Sorbello O, Moro MF, Cadoni F, Serra A, et al. The risk of bipolar disorders and major depressive disorders in Wilson disease: Results of a case control study. Int Clin Psychopharmacol. 2012;28:e61.
46. Zimbrean P, Seniow J. Cognitive and psychiatric symptoms in Wilson disease. Handb Clin Neurol. 2017;142:121–40.
47. Dening TR, Berrios GE. Wilson disease: a longitudinal study of psychiatric symptoms. Biol Psychiatry. 1990;28(3):255–65.
48. Svetel M, Potrebic A, Pekmezovic T, Tomic A, Kresojevic N, Jesic R, et al. Neuropsychiatric aspects of treated Wilson disease. Parkinsonism Relat Disord. 2009;15(10):772–5.
49. Dening TR, Berrios GE. Wilson disease. Psychiatric symptoms in 195 cases. Arch Gen Psychiatry. 1989;46(12):1126–34.
50. Sagawa M, Takao M, Nogawa S, Mizuno M, Murata M, Amano T, et al. Wilson disease associated with olfactory paranoid syn-

drome and idiopathic thrombocytopenic purpura. No To Shinkei. 2003;55(10):899–902.
51. Chung YS, Ravi SD, Borge GF. Psychosis in Wilson disease. Psychosomatics. 1986;27(1):65–6.
52. Shah N, Kumar D. Wilson disease, psychosis, and ECT. Convuls Ther. 1997;13(4):278–9.
53. Wichowicz HM, Cubala WJ, Slawek J. Wilson disease associated with delusional disorder. Psychiatry Clin Neurosci. 2006;60(6):758–60.
54. Huang CC, Chu NS. Wilson disease: clinical analysis of 71 cases and comparison with previous Chinese series. Journal of the Formosan Medical Association = Taiwan yi zhi. 1992;91(5):502–7.
55. Practice guideline for the assessment and treatment of patients with suicidal behaviors. Am J Psychiatry. 2003;160(11 Suppl):1–60.
56. Dening TR, Berrios GE. Wilson disease: a prospective study of psychopathology in 31 cases. Br J Psychiatry. 1989;155:206–13.
57. Freudenreich O, Holt DJ, Cather C, Goff DC. The evaluation and management of patients with first-episode schizophrenia: a selective, clinical review of diagnosis, treatment, and prognosis. Harv Rev Psychiatry. 2007;15(5):189–211.
58. EASL Clinical Practice Guidelines. Wilson disease. J Hepatol. 2012;56(3):671–85.
59. Cox DW. A screening test for Wilson disease and its application to psychiatric patients. Can Med Assoc J. 1967;96(2):83–6.
60. Gedack M, Schönfeldt-Lecuona C, Kratzer W, Kassubek J, Connemann B. P03-538 – ceruloplasmin serum concentrations in a randomized population sample of 2,445 subjects. Eur Psychiatry. 2011;26:1708.
61. Demily C, Parant F, Cheillan D, Broussolle E, Pavec A, Guillaud O, et al. Screening of Wilson disease in a psychiatric population: difficulties and pitfalls. A preliminary study. Ann General Psychiatry. 2017;16:19.
62. Brewer GJ. Wilson disease. In: Frucht SJFS, editor. Movement disorder emergencies: diagnosis and treatment. Totowa: Humana Press; 2007. p. 195–208.
63. Finelli PF. Kayser-Fleischer ring: hepatolenticular degeneration (Wilson disease). Neurology. 1995;45(7):1261–2.
64. Youn J, Kim JS, Kim HT, Lee JY, Lee PH, Ki CS, et al. Characteristics of neurological Wilson disease without Kayser-Fleischer ring. J Neurol Sci. 2012;323(1–2):183–6.

65. Herring NR, Konradi C. Myelin, copper, and the cuprizone model of schizophrenia. Front Biosci (Schol Ed). 2011;3:23–40.
66. Gonzalez-Estecha M, Trasobares EM, Tajima K, Cano S, Fernandez C, Lopez JL, et al. Trace elements in bipolar disorder. J Trace Elem Med Biol. 2011;25(Suppl 1):S78–83.
67. Bachmann H, Lossner J, Kuhn HJ, Biesold D, Siegemund R, Kunath B, et al. Long-term care and management of Wilson disease in the GDR. Eur Neurol. 1989;29(6):301–5.
68. Modai I, Karp L, Liberman UA, Munitz H. Penicillamine therapy for schizophreniform psychosis in Wilson disease. J Nerv Ment Dis. 1985;173(11):698–701.
69. Krim E, Barroso B. Psychiatric disorders treated with clozapine in a patient with Wilson disease. Presse Med. 2001;30(15):738.
70. Kulaksizoglu IB, Polat A. Quetiapine for mania with Wilson disease. Psychosomatics. 2003;44(5):438–9.
71. Kontaxakis V, Stefanis C, Markidis M, Tserpe V. Neuroleptic malignant syndrome in a patient with Wilson disease. J Neurol Neurosurg Psychiatry. 1988;51(7):1001–2.
72. Chroni E, Lekka NP, Tsibri E, Economou A, Paschalis C. Acute, progressive akinetic-rigid syndrome induced by neuroleptics in a case of Wilson disease. J Neuropsychiatry Clin Neurosci. 2001;13(4):531–2.
73. Bleakley S. Identifying and reducing the risk of antipsychotic drug interactions. Prog Neurol Psychiatry. 2012;16(2):20–4.
74. Woerwag-Mehta S, Hindley P, Hedderly T, Dhawan A. Complex psychiatric presentation in adolescent onset Wilson disease. BMJ Case Rep. 2011;2011 http//casereports.bmj.com/content/2011/bcr.01.2010.2628.full.pdf
75. Loganathan S, Nayak R, Sinha S, Taly AB, Math S, Varghese M. Treating mania in Wilson disease with lithium. J Neuropsychiatry Clin Neurosci. 2008;20(4):487–9.
76. Vaishnav P, Gandhi HA. Electro Convulsive Therapy in Psychiatric Manifestations in Wilson disease. Indian J Psychol Med. 2013;35(2):206–8.
77. Walter G, Lyndon B. Depression in hepatolenticular degeneration (Wilson disease). Aust N Z J Psychiatry. 1997;31(6):880–2.
78. Gill HH, Shankaran K, Desai HG. Wilson disease: varied hepatic presentations. Indian J Gastroenterol. 1994;13(3):95–8.
79. Knott A, Dieperink E, Willenbring ML, Heit S, Durfee JM, Wingert M, et al. Integrated psychiatric/medical care in a chronic hepatitis C clinic: effect on antiviral treatment evaluation and outcomes. Am J Gastroenterol. 2006;101(10):2254–62.

80. Minden SL, Ding L, Cleary PD, Frankel D, Glanz BI, Healy BC, et al. Improving the quality of mental health care in multiple sclerosis. J Neurol Sci. 2013;335(1–2):42–7.
81. Wilson Disease Centers of Excellence. Available from: https://www.wilsonsdisease.org/for-patients-families/centers-of-excellence
82. Sorbello O, Riccio D, Sini M, Carta M, Demelia L. Resolved Psychosis after liver transplantation in a patient with Wilson disease. Clin Pract Epidemiol Ment Health. 2011;7:182–4.
83. Lankarani KB, Malek-Hosseini SA, Nikeghbalian S, Dehghani M, Pourhashemi M, Kazemi K, et al. Fourteen years of experience of liver transplantation for Wilson disease; a report on 107 cases from Shiraz, Iran. PLoS One. 2016;11(12):e0167890.
84. Al-Hilou H, Hebbar S, Gunson BK, Claridge LC, Syn WK, Holt AP. Long term outcomes of liver transplantation for Wilson disease: a single centre experience. Gut. 2012;61:A210.
85. Geissler I, Heinemann K, Rohm S, Hauss J, Lamesch P. Liver transplantation for hepatic and neurological Wilson disease. Transplant Proc. 2003;35(4):1445–6.
86. Stracciari A, Tempestini A, Borghi A, Guarino M. Effect of liver transplantation on neurological manifestations in Wilson disease. Arch Neurol. 2000;57(3):384–6.

Chapter 8
Monitoring Treatment of Wilson Disease

Tamir Miloh and Michael L. Schilsky

Monitoring for Effectiveness of Treatment

Treatment of WD in an asymptomatic patient aims to prevent the development or progression of signs and symptoms of disease. In symptomatic patients, the goal is to achieve stabilization and improvement of signs and symptoms of disease. Monitoring is the means by which we determine if these goals are met. Monitoring for effectiveness utilizes clinical parameters (symptoms and physical exam for signs of disease), laboratory testing (blood and urine and in some liver biopsy), and assessment of adherence with

T. Miloh
Pediatric Hepatology and Liver Transplant Medicine, Texas Children's Hospital, Houston, TX, USA

Baylor College of Medicine, Houston, TX, USA
e-mail: tamiloh@texaschildrens.org

M. L. Schilsky (✉)
Division of Digestive Diseases and Transplant and Immunology, Departments of Medicine and Surgery, Yale University, New Haven, CT, USA
e-mail: michael.schilsky@yale.edu

M. L. Schilsky (ed.), *Management of Wilson Disease*, Clinical Gastroenterology, https://doi.org/10.1007/978-3-319-91527-2_8

Table 8.1 Monitoring of patients with Wilson disease

Clinical evaluation history	Hepatic, neurologic, and psychiatric assessment	Every visit
Physical exam	Focus on chronic liver disease and neurologic exam, mental health testing if appropriate history obtained	Every visit
Blood test	CBC with platelets, PT/INR, liver panel, serum copper, and ceruloplasmin	Every 6 months for maintenance therapy, more frequent during treatment initiation and to follow abnormal results
Urine tests	Urinalysis, 24-h urine collection for copper (also zinc for patients on Zn)	At least every 6 months, after changes in treatment
Adherence	Discuss adherence and any barriers to adherence, assess by clinical and biochemical parameters, input from pharmacies about refills	Every visit
Scoring systems	Child-Pugh-Turcotte and MELD-Na, (in those with cirrhosis) modified Nazer (in those with liver failure), UWDRS or equivalent for tracking neurologic disease	As clinically indicated
Medication side effects	Look for neurologic or psychiatric worsening, dyspepsia, bone marrow suppression, nephropathy, arthropathy, skin changes	Every visit

Table 8.1 (continued)

Overtreatment (in patients on long-term therapy)	Neuropathy, low white cell count and thrombocytopenia, lower serum and urine copper, and reduced ceruloplasmin	At least every 6 months
Dietary adherence	Ask about dietary copper restriction	Every visit, consultation with registered dietician at caregiver or patient request

Liver panel = ALT, AST, alkaline phosphatase, total and direct bilirubin, GGTP

medications and diet. A summary of monitoring labs is given in Table 8.1 [1]. To some degree, monitoring is tailored to each patient's clinical status, degree of hepatic, neurologic and psychiatric disease, and special needs, but there are common elements that help us determine if treatment is successful. The frequency of monitoring is higher during the initial phase of initiation of medical therapy and can be less frequent once disease stabilization is achieved, which is hereafter referred to as the maintenance phase. Patients are encouraged to use tools such as the Lab Tracker (see the Wilson Disease Association Website for download) to help maintain records of their monitoring that can be reviewed with their health-care providers. In this chapter, we will review the different aspects of monitoring of treatment of patients with WD.

Monitoring: Visit Frequency

During the first year of therapy, patients should be seen by their health-care providers and undergo laboratory testing at least every 3 months and afterward at 6-month intervals. Patients with decompensated cirrhosis or unstable neurologic or psychiatric symptoms may need to be seen and monitored more frequently, weekly or twice monthly, while the dosage of medication is increased to goal, and it is clear medications are being tolerated, or when medical treatments are changed. Once the patients' disease becomes more stable, visit and testing frequently may be decreased. If there is evidence or suspicion of nonadherence to treatment, patients may be seen more frequently, and assistance from family and other providers, counselors, or pharmacists is sought to try to improve this problem [2].

Monitoring: Clinical Examination

The aim of clinical examinations by health-care providers differs in asymptomatic and symptomatic patients. In asymptomatic patients, the examination should focus on confirming the lack of any signs of liver disease, neurologic disease, or psychiatric symptoms. In symptomatic patients, there are unique areas to focus on, including signs of liver, neurologic, or psychiatric disease. Careful attention to history as well as physical examination is important for each of these categories. For instance, a new history of darkening urine, generalized itching (pruritus), or easy bruising may indicate the presence of liver disease. For children who are in school, a decline in school performance may indicate signs of cognitive change or of mood disturbance. Similarly, in adults, falls may indicate changes in coordination or balance and increase suspicion of neurologic disease, while a disruption of personal relationships may be a sign of a mood disorder, all possibly related to WD.

With respect to clinical signs of liver disease seen on examination, new onset of jaundice and scleral icterus (yellowing of the conjunctiva of the eyes), excoriations from pruritus, bruises from a low platelet count and coagulation defect, the appearance of ascites, or signs of hepatic encephalopathy (altered mentation, tremor or flapping tremor known as asterixis) may indicate disease worsening and progressive liver disease [3].

With appropriate medical therapy over time, many of the signs and symptoms of liver dysfunction are expected to improve. Therefore monitoring must take into account what signs and symptoms were present, and these must be followed over time. The initial response to treatment should be disease stabilization, but over time further improvement often occurs. However for patients with very advanced liver disease and decompensated cirrhosis, though a trial of therapy may be warranted, a referral to a transplant center for evaluation for liver transplant is also appropriate [4]. Some with advanced disease with jaundice, pruritus and bleeding (due to coagulopathy), or ascites may improve over time on medical therapy. Initially patients with ascites may find it easier to control the ascites, and medical treatments such as diuretics may be reduced or even stopped when the ascites is resolved. For those with varices and bleeding, there may be a reduction in size of the varices. Hepatic encephalopathy may also become easier to control or resolve altogether as treatment takes effect and liver function improves [1].

For those with Kayser-Fleischer (KF) rings due to WD, these resolve with treatment, but the rate of their disappearance may vary with the treatment and the size of the ring at time of initiation of treatment (larger and concentric rings would take longer to disappear than faint rings only found superiorly and inferiorly on the cornea) and may not reflect the rate of change in neurologic or psychiatric symptoms if these are present. Similarly, the rare finding of sunflowcr cataracts also may improve with treatment aimed at copper removal. In patients without KF rings or sunflower cataracts, their appearance may reflect disease worsening or nonadherence. Similarly, nonadherence should be suspected in those with KF rings that become larger with time on serial examination [1].

Neurologic symptoms may exacerbate with the initiation of chelation in a minority of patients, and in these individuals, there may be progression of tremor and increased muscle tone (dystonia) leading to at times painful contractures and even fixed deformity. In most however, the initial symptoms that are present may improve with time; however some may develop fixed changes and permanent disability [5]. Patients with neurologic signs or symptoms should see a neurologist at the outset of their disease to be able to track their progress on treatment and also treat any neurologic symptoms. There are some validated scales that have been used to define the degree of neurologic impairment. One such example is the Unified Wilson Disease Rating Scale (UWDRS), a scoring system developed by neurologists to help give an objective score to the degree of neurologic impairment in WD [6]. Use of the UWDRS is mostly for clinical trials where tracking is mostly for clinical trials where tracking of improvements in the score would indicate neurologic disease due to WD is improving. Practically, patients' caregivers may take a video of the patient doing a specific activity at home and then repeat this over time doing the same activity. In addition, comparison of the ability of the patient over time to do daily tasks helps gauge the degree of improvement in their disease [7]. Monitoring neurologic or psychiatric signs and symptoms in WD is complex and discussed in a different chapter. The UWDRS was developed to standardize the clinical assessment of neurologic involvement in patients with WD and is mostly used for clinical studies.

Psychiatric symptoms may be present at the outset and often precede the establishment of the diagnosis of WD. They may be as subtle as emotional mood swings to full-blown depression and psychosis. If they are absent at the start, their appearance in well-treated patients often indicates nonadherence with treatment or underlying psychiatric disease that could occur independent of WD or be worsened by WD. In many who develop symptomatic disease, there may be improvement with treatment of their WD, but careful attention to patient's symptoms is important, and pharmacologic treatment of the psychiatric symptoms may improve the patient's status [8].

Monitoring: Laboratory Testing

Biochemical monitoring of patients with WD includes blood and urine testing. Liver biopsy with histology and copper quantitation is most often a one-time event at time of diagnosis, and serial biopsy and evaluation are only needed when there is a question of treatment failure or a secondary liver injury or disease as well as WD.

Blood testing for monitoring includes complete blood count (CBC) and platelets, liver tests, and coagulation parameters. Often a comprehensive profile that includes electrolytes and liver tests is ordered, and this enables tracking of kidney function as well.

Blood counts should be monitored at regular intervals as noted above or more frequently if there are abnormalities. A low value for hemoglobin on the CBC may be a marker of non-autoimmune hemolytic anemia, most often in untreated patients or in patients with acute liver failure. Specific testing can be ordered to determine if this is present, including a blood smear to look for cells with signs of hemolysis and other biochemical markers of hemolysis such as haptoglobin. However a low hemoglobin, or anemia, can occur with iron deficiency or due to other causes such as bone marrow suppression from medications or toxic agents [1]. In long-term treated patients, anemia can be due to overtreatment and a relatively low copper state for the bone marrow. In this setting, tests such as ferritin that reflect tissue iron are elevated, and biopsy of bone marrow or liver will show excess iron stores [9].

Low white blood cell count (WBC) can be a marker of portal hypertension but can also occur due to bone marrow suppression from D-penicillamine. Low WBC can also be found in copper deficiency and is seen in WD patients with overtreatment with any agent. With current therapies, this typically does not occur for years after treatment is initiated.

Low platelets (thrombocytopenia below 150,000) are marker of progressive portal hypertension but can also be a marker of bone marrow suppression from treatment for WD (D-penicillamine or trientine) or overtreatment after time on any therapy [10]. With respect to worsening portal hypertension, lower platelet counts accompanied by new splenomegaly, ascites, or varices (seen on endoscopy) portend treatment failure, and this is discussed below. When there is no gross evidence of advanced liver disease as seen by signs of portal hypertension, then the degree of liver fibrosis can also be estimated and used for monitoring. There are some useful serum tests that can be applied, APRI score and FIB-4 [11], but also types of liver imaging known as elastography can be helpful as well (discussed below).

Liver enzymes, ALT and AST, typically normalize over the first 6–18 months of treatment. Some liver tests in patients with advanced liver disease may not normalize but should improve and stabilize. Persistently abnormal liver enzymes (more than twice upper limit of normal) may be a marker of underdosing, nonadherence, treatment failure, or secondary liver injury [12]. Dose adjustment, assessing adherence, or alternative therapy should be considered. Normalization of liver enzymes is expected to reduce the risk of fibrosis progression. Total bilirubin may be elevated with hemolysis, and increased direct bilirubin is a marker of liver dysfunction. Coagulopathy (INR) often improves with chelation and correction of vitamin K deficiency (which may be common in patients with cholestasis). Levels of serum albumin are expected to improve with therapy and nutrition. Electrolytes, in particular renal function, should be monitored, as some chelation therapy may be associated with nephrotoxicity. Patients on D-penicillamine and trientine should have monitoring with urinalysis to monitor nephropathy (nephritis and proteinuria) [1].

Although serum transaminases (ALT and AST) are referred to as liver tests, they really are markers of liver injury. Albumin and INR are markers of the true function of liver cells; however albumin is influenced by inflammation (it is a negative acute phase marker), by nutritional state (low in malnourished states), and when there is loss of albumin from the kidney (proteinuria) or from the gut (in protein-losing enteropathy). Therefore following the international normalized prothrombin time (PT) or INR reflects liver function more directly, with some exceptions. There are vitamin K-dependent factors that make up the coagulation cascade that is measured by the PT, and in states with vitamin K deficiency as can occur if there is prolonged elevated bilirubin (cholestasis), then PT and INR is elevated. In those individuals, INR after vitamin K replacement will represent true liver function and coagulation status better. Other rare clotting disorders also can give elevation in PT and INR without indicating liver dysfunction, but these are extremely rare. Therefore elevation of INR in a patient with WD indicates hepatic synthetic dysfunction and is a parameter that can be followed with time to show healing with treatment [13]. Other clinical scores that can be monitored in a patient without acute presentation include PELD (patients younger than 12 years of age), MELD (for patients older than 12), and the Child-Pugh scores.

Monitoring: Copper Status

Copper levels can be measured in the blood and urine and liver tissue. While routine monitoring of liver copper is not typical due to the need to perform liver biopsy for this measurement, monitoring of copper status using parameters from blood and urine is important to evaluate response to therapy, adjust medication dosing, and assess nonadherence to therapy. Nonceruloplasmin copper (NCC), sometimes referred to as "free copper" in the circulation, is an important marker of copper status. NCC can be estimated by measuring total serum copper (mcg/dl) directly and subtracting from this the estimated amount of copper in the protein ceruloplasmin (calculated using the serum level of ceruloplasmin (mg/dl) times 3.15). Before treatment, especially in symptomatic patients, NCC is typically higher than 15 mcg/dl. With treatment patients should have values between 5 and 15 mcg/dl. Patients who are nonadherent with medication or dietary copper content and who had a normal range NCC will often have a higher value when retested for this estimation. On the other end of the spectrum are those who are over treated. These individuals will have levels below 5 mcg/dl, often with accompanying changes in their blood counts (low white blood cell count and anemia).

In about 20% of patients, commercial assays for measurement of copper and ceruloplasmin do not give a positive value for NCC, and in these patients, it is not very useful to follow this estimated value. In this instance, measurements of urine copper and following liver tests and blood counts may be the only way to characterize their copper status and treatment effectiveness. More accurate methods to monitor efficacy by standard copper and copper protein analysis remain to be developed [1].

Urine copper excretion is thought to mirror NCC as urine copper is derived from this exchangeable blood component. Urine copper excretion over 24 h is commonly used as a measurement for copper status. Single "spot" measurements do not reflect the true overall copper balance and may lead to under- or overestimates for an individual. Twenty-four-hour urine copper is typically elevated above 100 mcg at the time of diagnosis and before treatment in symptomatic patients. In asymptomatic patients and some younger patients with silent liver disease, the value may not reach diagnostic levels of 100 mcg/day and may even be within the upper limits of the normal range. With introduction of chelation therapy with D-penicillamine or trientine, urine copper may initially increase to more than 1000 mcg/24 h, as renal excretion is the mode of copper elimination with these drugs. Over time, urine 24 h copper excretion decreases to about 150–250 mcg daily in patients on maintenance doses of trientine and 250–500 mcg for those on maintenance D-penicillamine treatment. In patients on zinc therapy, the 24-h urine excretion of copper decreases with treatment if it was elevated at the start, as the mode of action is decreased intestinal copper absorption and urine copper excretion in these patients reflects the status of their NCC [2]. Shown in Table 8.2 are treatment goals for urine copper excretion for each treatment discussed above.

Monitoring: Liver and Brain Imaging

An ultrasound or sonogram is a useful baseline test for any patient with WD. At times, it is also helpful to perform a Doppler study of the blood flow through the liver to exclude any blockage of flow in the portal or hepatic vein and look at hepatic arterial blood flow. A Doppler study is typically done

TABLE 8.2 Urine copper excretion (micrograms for 24 h) on treatment for Wilson disease

Treatment	Treatment goal	Initial treatment	Undertreatment or nonadherence	Overtreatment or nonadherence
Penicillamine	250–500	>1000	>500	<150
Trientine	150–250	>1000	>500	<100
Zinc	30–120	30–120	>120 (or trend upward from baseline)	<30

at the same time as the ultrasound of the liver. The presence of an enlarged spleen along with ascites or change in the liver shape may suggest cirrhosis is present. For patients with earlier stage liver disease, an ultrasound can also suggest the presence of fatty change that may be present at the outset due to WD but also can occur in patients with fatty liver disease or after alcohol use. More advanced imaging, CT or MR, and even MR spectroscopy can be used to estimate the degree of fatty liver. Alternatively the amount of fatty change can be estimated on liver biopsy. In most patients with fatty change in the liver due to WD, the fat deposition decreases with treatment and the above modes of liver imaging can often be used to look for this improvement. In those where the fatty change in the liver is independent of the WD, this will not resolve.

The standard for evaluating and demonstrating progression of liver fibrosis is by liver biopsy; however there are now noninvasive imaging methods for estimating the amount of hepatic fibrosis. Examples of technology to measure fibrosis noninvasively include sonographic methods using sound waves (acoustic radiation force elastography or Fibroscan™) and MR elastography (MRE). There are few validated studies for these methods for WD, but their use in general liver practice has been increasing [11, 14, 15].

Initial screening and surveillance for primary liver cancer, HCC, should be performed in cirrhotic patients with WD. Imaging for routine surveillance should be by ultrasound; however when abnormalities are seen on ultrasound, dynamic imaging with CT or MRI with contrast is needed. Surveillance imaging is typically done on a 6-month basis; however when abnormalities are seen and closer follow-up is warranted, then the follow-up studies often are recommended at 3 months' time [16].

When there is identification of abnormal brain MRI or CT seen on the initial imaging, it may be useful to obtain a follow-up study if there is clinical change, especially if there is worsening. Usually, repeat brain imaging is something that a neurologist would request in the course of their assessment [17, 18].

Monitoring: Defining and Monitoring for Treatment Failure

Treatment failure for patients on therapy with WD can be assessed by progression or lack of improvement in patients' symptoms, laboratory tests (liver tests, coagulation, and copper parameters), or intolerable side effects of medications or safety concerns [1]. In one retrospective study in Europe, the presence of liver tests (ALT and AST) that are twice the baseline value or more than that after treatment for a time (typically beyond 3–6 months) would be considered a possible treatment failure and dose changes or alteration in therapy considered [19]. For copper parameters, failure to improve NCC and urinary copper to desired goals should prompt a look at patient adherence and diet. If both of these have been good, then changes in therapy are appropriate [1].

With respect to side effects from the medications, these may range from laboratory abnormalities to clinical findings and symptoms or both. Changes in therapy for patients on D-penicillamine due to side effects can range up to about 25–30% of patients, less frequent on trientine [10]. Zinc does not cause known lab abnormalities other than an elevation in pancreatic amylase or lipase without any true pancreatitis (either by symptoms or imaging) [2].

Treatment would be considered as failing in patients on therapy with serious clinical deterioration such as the development of jaundice in a patient without this sign, persisting jaundice in a patient with jaundice after treatment, or worsening signs and symptoms of portal hypertension such as a new onset of ascites, upper GI bleeding due to varices, hepatic encephalopathy, or change in kidney function due to hepatorenal syndrome. For patients with cirrhosis of the liver, the Child-Pugh-Turcotte status or MELD-Na score can be assessed, and rising scores indicate a failed response to therapy. These patients then need to be urgently referred for liver transplantation while maintained on treatment if possible [1]. The modified Wilson disease score can also guide on treatment failure for those patients with severe hepatic disease or acute liver failure at the outset [20]. A rising score, even if below the threshold of 10 below which medical therapy is thought to work most of the time, should prompt more frequent observation and close tracking of the patient. A continued rising score would be considered treatment failure.

Monitoring: Overtreatment of WD

Overtreatment for WD (over chelation) can present with symptomatic copper deficiency including hematological side effects such as anemia and neutropenia and neurological symptoms including sensory or motor-sensory neuropathies and myelopathies which normally reverse with correction of the deficiency if detected in time. Monitoring for overtreatment is important on all treatments for WD and can be diagnosed by low NCC and 24-h urine copper [9, 21].

Adherence should be monitored with every visit as it is key in the long-term follow-up of patients with WD and is lifelong after diagnosis. Nonadherence may lead to acute hepatitis, hepatic failure, neuropsychiatric deterioration, and ultimately death [22]. Nonadherence has been reported in more than 50% of the patients, in particular those without overt symptoms. Ongoing monitoring of medication intake significantly contributed to total and partial improvements of symptoms, self-assessment of well-being, and decreased risk of clinical deterioration. Self-report and physician assessment of adherence have its limitations and are not always accurate. Evidence of nonadherence includes appearance or reappearance of Kayser-Fleischer rings, fluctuating liver enzymes, elevated NCC, and increased or decreased 24-h urinary copper (depending on treatment). Adherence in WD patients taking zinc can be confirmed by urinary zinc excretion >2 mg/24 h, though this only demonstrates the use of zinc around the time of the treatment. Another measure to follow adherence is by appropriate pharmacy refills; however this may be complicated by changing insurances and use of multiple pharmacies. Barriers to nonadherence should be addressed. These include medications' side effects, complexity of regimen, cost, and limited access [1]. Cognitive impairment and lower executive functioning were documented in some patients with WD, particularly patients with neurologic symptoms, and this can affect adherence as well. The presence of psychiatric symptoms such as depression may also result in lower adherence. A neuropsychological assessment may be valuable to assess the presence and consequences of cognitive impairments or psychiatric symptoms that may be a target for intervention [23]. Adherence to a low copper diet may be challenging for a few patients and is further discussed in the nutrition chapter. The dietary restrictions on copper should be stricter within the first year of therapy, especially in symptomatic patients. Consultation with a dietitian is advisable for individual patients and families. Patients with suspected nonadherence should be monitored more frequently.

Conclusions

Monitoring of treatment for WD is important for determining treatment efficacy and safety. Monitoring should be more frequent around initiation of therapy in symptomatic patients but should continue at regular intervals after for maintenance therapy. Monitoring includes clinical examination, blood and urine testing, and imaging of the liver or brain when appropriate. Parameters that are used to assess copper status, estimation of NCC, and 24-h urine copper determinations should be followed over time. Monitoring and measures to address barriers to good adherence to medication and diet should be performed over time. Changes of therapy should follow treatment failure or identification of safety issues. Overtreatment that necessitates holding of current WD treatment or dose reduction of medication can be identified by changes in copper status, presence of a new low WBC or anemia that is not due to iron deficiency, or appearance of new neurologic symptoms. Lifelong care monitoring is required for the treatment of WD and is best accomplished by a partnership between patient and their health-care providers. The use of tools that help patients track their monitoring, such as the lab tracker, aids in this process and can facilitate discussion between patients and providers.

References

1. Roberts EA, Schilsky ML, American D, Association for Study of Liver. *Diagnosis and treatment of Wilson disease: an update*. Hepatology. 2008;47(6):2089–111.
2. Schilsky ML. Wilson disease: diagnosis, treatment, and follow-up. Clin Liver Dis. 2017;21(4):755–67.
3. Wong RJ, et al. A clinical assessment of Wilson disease in patients with concurrent liver disease. J Clin Gastroenterol. 2011;45(3):267–73.
4. Beinhardt S, et al. Long-term outcomes of patients with Wilson disease in a large Austrian cohort. Clin Gastroenterol Hepatol. 2014;12(4):683–9.
5. Litwin T, et al. Early neurological worsening in patients with Wilson's disease. J Neurol Sci. 2015;355(1–2):162–7.
6. Czlonkowska A, et al. Unified Wilson's disease rating scale – a proposal for the neurological scoring of Wilson's disease patients. Neurol Neurochir Pol. 2007;41(1):1–12.
7. Leinweber B, et al. Evaluation of the unified Wilson's disease rating scale (UWDRS) in German patients with treated Wilson's disease. Mov Disord. 2008;23(1):54–62.
8. Mura G, et al. Psychiatric comorbidity in Wilson's disease. Int Rev Psychiatry. 2017;29(5):445–62.
9. Willis MS, et al. Zinc-induced copper deficiency: a report of three cases initially recognized on bone marrow examination. Am J Clin Pathol. 2005;123(1):125–31.
10. Weiss KH, et al. Efficacy and safety of oral chelators in treatment of patients with Wilson disease. Clin Gastroenterol Hepatol. 2013;11(8):1028-35 e1-2.
11. Karlas T, et al. Non-invasive evaluation of hepatic manifestation in Wilson disease with transient elastography, ARFI, and different fibrosis scores. Scand J Gastroenterol. 2012;47(11):1353–61.
12. Iorio R, et al. Serum transaminases in children with Wilson's disease. J Pediatr Gastroenterol Nutr. 2004;39(4):331–6.

13. Dhawan A, et al. Wilson's disease in children: 37-year experience and revised King's score for liver transplantation. Liver Transpl. 2005;11(4):441–8.
14. Sini M, et al. Non-invasive assessment of hepatic fibrosis in a series of patients with Wilson's disease. Dig Liver Dis. 2012;44(6):487–91.
15. Sinha S, et al. Sequential MRI changes in Wilson's disease with de-coppering therapy: a study of 50 patients. Br J Radiol. 2007;80(957):744–9.
16. Boga S, Ala A, Schilsky ML. Hepatic features of Wilson disease. Handb Clin Neurol. 2017;142:91–9.
17. Czlonkowska A, Litwin T, Chabik G. Wilson disease: neurologic features. Handb Clin Neurol. 2017;142:101–19.
18. Kim TJ, et al. MR imaging of the brain in Wilson disease of childhood: findings before and after treatment with clinical correlation. AJNR Am J Neuroradiol. 2006;27(6):1373–8.
19. Weiss KH, et al. Zinc monotherapy is not as effective as chelating agents in treatment of Wilson disease. Gastroenterology. 2011;140(4):1189–1198 e1.
20. Nazer H, et al. Wilson's disease: clinical presentation and use of prognostic index. Gut. 1986;27(11):1377–81.
21. Dziezyc K, et al. Symptomatic copper deficiency in three Wilson's disease patients treated with zinc sulphate. Neurol Neurochir Pol. 2014;48(3):214–8.
22. Dziezyc K, et al. Compliant treatment with anti-copper agents prevents clinically overt Wilson's disease in pre-symptomatic patients. Eur J Neurol. 2014;21(2):332–7.
23. Wenisch E, et al. Cognitive profile in Wilson's disease: a case series of 31 patients. Rev Neurol (Paris). 2013;169(12):944–9.

Chapter 9
Unique Pediatric Aspects of Wilson Disease

Michelle Camarata and Regino P. Gonzalez-Peralta

Introduction

Overall, WD is a rare cause of liver disease in childhood. However, children and adolescents comprise a considerable proportion of patients that present with WD [1, 2]. In this

---

Disclosures Dr. Gonzalez-Peralta is on advisory boards for Genentech-Roche, Kadmon, and Shire and scientific board of the Wilson Disease Association; he also receives grant support from Gilead, AbbVie, and Merck.

M. Camarata
Department of Gastroenterology and Hepatology, Royal Surrey County Hospital, Guildford, Surrey, UK

Department of Clinical and Experimental Medicine, University of Surrey, Guildford, Surrey, UK

Department of Surgery, Section of Transplant and Immunology, Yale School of Medicine, New Haven, CT, USA

R. P. Gonzalez-Peralta (✉)
Division of Pediatric Gastroenterology, Hepatology and Liver Transplantation, Florida Hospital for Children, Orlando, FL, USA
e-mail: Regino.Gonzalez-Peralta.MD@flhosp.org

M. L. Schilsky (ed.), *Management of Wilson Disease*, Clinical Gastroenterology, https://doi.org/10.1007/978-3-319-91527-2_9

regard, it is interesting to point out that all patients originally described by Dr. Wilson were young when they initially became symptomatic [3]. Although rare, clinically apparent WD in infants within the first year of life is increasingly recognized [4–6]. Therefore, WD should be considered in those with suggestive symptoms or biochemical abnormalities regardless of age. Assessing for WD through prenatal testing, at birth, or in asymptomatic first-degree relatives of patients with WD may reduce the age of diagnosis by early identification of presymptomatic patients. Early identification is critically important as it results in the timely institution of treatment and a more favorable outcome than in those who are identified late [7–10].

As commonly occurs in pediatrics, a major challenge in identifying and managing children with WD is the relative paucity of age-specific data to inform practitioners about best therapies. There are only a few small-sized studies that describe WD exclusively in children. However, the diagnosis, treatment, and monitoring guidelines for WD as carefully detailed for adults in other chapters elsewhere in this handbook are generally applicable for children. A clinical position statement on WD in children was also recently published [11]. In the following we highlight some salient features of WD that we consider unique to children.

Diagnosis

Wilson disease predominantly presents clinically with hepatic or neuropsychiatric symptoms or commonly some combination of these. Most children with WD present with liver dysfunction [12, 13]. In general, approximately 50% of children (less than 18 years old) and up to 75% of those less than 10 years old present with liver disease [14]. It is likely that this is related to the natural history of WD as copper presumably accumulates first in the liver. Some have speculated that in addition, the predominance of hepatic presentation may be linked to the presence of gene deletion mutations that are associated with early-onset disease [12, 13]. As for adults, the spectrum of liver disease in children and adolescents varies widely from asymptomatic derangement of biochemical liver tests (most common) to chronic hepatic disease – cirrhosis to acute liver failure. Hematological, endocrinological, and other abnormalities are infrequently the initial findings at presentation of WD in childhood [14].

Although hepatic presentation of WD is most common in childhood, it is critically important to avoid overlooking the disease in young patients with neuropsychiatric symptoms, particularly those that arise rather suddenly. These symptoms may include neurologic symptoms typically found in adults with WD, like speech difficulties, drooling, and tremors. However, changes such as worsening handwriting can be subtle and easily missed until it is severe. Some symptoms may be too non-specific to attract much parental attention. For example, gait incoordination may be ascribed to simple clumsiness or athletic inaptitude rather than to a primary neurologic problem. Psychiatric symptoms may include difficulty with concentration and memory resulting in deteriorating academic performance in school that may be perceived as laziness or irresponsible childhood behavior. Depression, withdrawal, and antisocial and other abnormal behaviors, particularly in adolescents, may be ascribed as "normal" for age or related to social stressors and not psychiatric disease.

As in adults, the diagnosis of WD in children depends on a composite of clinical features and specific laboratory, histological, and genetic test results. The diagnosis of WD can be particularly challenging in the very young child [15]. Several aspects of data interpretation and sample collection are unique to the pediatric population and can be particularly challenging in this group.

Kayser-Fleischer (KF) rings, a yellow-brown pigmentation in the periphery of the cornea, represent abnormal copper deposition in this structure's Descemet's membrane. Kayser-Fleischer rings can support the diagnosis of WD but are often absent in children. When they are present, these rings first arise as an arc in the superior pole of the cornea and then in its inferior pole, and finally with persistent copper accumulation, the arcs link to complete the ring. Kayser-Fleischer rings are occasionally present on simple eye examination but are most often only visible on slit-lamp assessment by an experienced practitioner [16]. Pediatric series suggest that overall, they occur in some 40% of children with WD (range 14–88%) [17]. It should be highlighted that the absence of KF rings does not exclude the diagnosis of WD. However, when present, particularly in those with neuropsychiatric symptoms, it strongly suggests the diagnosis of WD and should expeditiously prompt further investigation. Of note, KF rings are not unique to WD and can be seen rarely in other chronic cholestatic diseases and cirrhosis where secondary copper accumulation leads to corneal deposition of this metal.

Elevated 24-h urinary copper excretion can be useful in establishing the diagnosis of WD, but in asymptomatic children with WD, the urine copper may be normal. Contamination of the urine sample and incomplete collections can affect the accuracy of the result for 24-h urine copper testing and hinder its interpretation. Hence, strict precautions during the collection process need to be taken that can be particularly challenging in infants and young children. To minimize potential problems, urine collection should be undertaken on a dedicated day without distractions, trips, or other planned activities. The use of urine "hats" under toilets can be especially useful for collection in girls. Collecting samples from babies may involve the use of a special bag attached to the skin with adhesive tape and a diaper placed over the bag. The infant will need to be monitored often and the sample bag changed and emptied into a dedicated container after each urination.

The penicillamine challenge test (PCT) was suggested as a way of improving the accuracy of the 24-h urine copper test in children [18]. In this modification of the test, D-penicillamine (a copper chelator) is administered at a dose of 500 mg at the start of the 24-h urine collection and midway through it, 12 h later. Urinary copper excretion of more than 1675 mg over 24 h after the challenge is considered suggestive of WD. However, further experience has provoked reassessment of the PCT [19]. For example, the frequency of falsely normal or elevated copper excretion with the D-penicillamine challenge and the lack of studies for this test in unaffected heterozygous carriers of WD limit the interpretation of its true sensitivity and specificity [20]. A subsequent pediatric study suggested that PCT was of little use to diagnose WD in asymptomatic children with abnormal liver tests [21].

Low serum ceruloplasmin level is another important diagnostic marker of WD. Although normal ceruloplasmin concentration is stable for adults, it considerably varies with age in children: from very low during infancy through the first 6 months of life (less than 10 mg/dL) to peak levels in early childhood (30–50 mg/mL) before settling in the adult range (greater than 20 mg/dL) [22]. Thus, interpreting results of serum ceruloplasmin concentration in children requires careful appraisal.

If the diagnosis of WD remains uncertain with blood and urine tests, a liver biopsy may be necessary. A percutaneous liver biopsy is a procedure where a small tissue sample is collected using a needle inserted through the skin and into the liver. The liver tissue is fixed and prepared for examination under a microscope, and its concentration of copper can be determined from a sample as well. To perform the procedure safely, children usually require sedation or anesthesia. Although liver biopsy is safe, major complications such as bleeding requiring transfusion, surgery, or intensive care management and chest complications including, pneumothorax or hemothorax, occur uncommonly [23, 24]. Nicastro et al. (2010) noted a significant difference between hepatic copper in children with WD and unaffected controls [21]. These investigators noted liver copper levels less than 75 micrograms (μg)/gram of dry weight (gdw) in only 2/30 (7%) of pediatric patients with WD and greater than 50 μg/gdw in only 4/24 (6%) controls. Thus, these investigators proposed a hepatic copper concentration threshold of 75 μg/gdw as optimal to diagnose WD in children [21, 25].

Delivering distressing news about the diagnosis of a lifelong illness such as WD is always difficult, particularly when the patient is a child. In addition, the pediatric practitioner is always faced with dealing with several "patients" simultaneously (the affected child or adolescent, their parents, and potentially other relatives). To ensure success, all interested close family members need to be involved in these discussions during which complex information is conveyed in an age-appropriate manner. Having these important discussions in a private, child-friendly space other than the usual examination room may be best as such places may put the child and family at greatest ease. It is important to avoid underestimating a young child's ability to understand, and therefore health team members must remain vigilant about body language and facial expressions, as these sometimes say more than plain words. Initially, assess the child's knowledge, often repeat information, and avoid long explanations. The use of diagrams and other age-appropriate visual cues may be helpful aids to improve understanding and keep the child engaged. After initial discussions, ascertain the child and parent's understanding of what has been explained. Children may need extra time to understand and process the diagnosis, treatment, and monitoring plans. Be prepared to answer the same questions on repeated occasions. Listen to the ideas, concerns, and expectations of the patient-family nucleus. Because it may be difficult for patients and relatives to fully comprehend all of the information during an initial discussion, unanswered questions or concerns should be sought at subsequent follow-up visits.

Older children and adolescents may be particularly vulnerable to perceptions of being different and may struggle with the potential impact of a chronic illness in their future. Innovative peer-group support mechanisms such as blogs, electronic apps, and social media support groups can be useful for helping older children and adolescents engage with patients in a similar age group with WD. Similarly, parents frequently feel guilty about having passed down a genetic disease. Because parents may perceive shame, they may withhold this information; hence, it is critically important for practitioners to actively strive to discuss these issues in a nonjudgmental manner, particularly during initial visits. Practitioners should encourage parents to seek support from community resources such as church, a social group, or trained counselor. It is important for the child and parents to develop a dedicated support system. Alerting and educating individuals involved in the child's life, such as teachers, babysitters, and other parents, about WD may be helpful in ensuring successful management and in uncovering potential difficulties.

Treatment

Wilson disease treatment is lifelong, and compliance with the prescribed medical regimen is essential to prevent clinical progression and achieve a favorable outcome. As for adults, treatment options include oral chelators (trientine and D-penicillamine) and zinc salts. Chelators exert their therapeutic effect by binding to copper and increasing its urinary excretion, whereas zinc salts act by reducing intestinal copper absorption (see chapter on treatment of WD and below). In children, finding a tolerable drug and formulation is particularly important to enhance adherence. Cost and treatment availability may also dictate treatment options.

In symptomatic patients with WD, trientine is as effective and probably has fewer side effects than D-penicillamine; therefore, it is becoming the preferred initial treatment, when available. Accumulating pediatric-specific data suggests that trientine is safe and effective in children with WD [26, 27]. As is generally common in pediatric practice, dosage in children is weight based (20 mg/kg/day for both trientine and D-penicillamine, divided into at least two doses) [17]. As such, dosing needs careful appraisal during follow-up and is progressively adjusted with normal childhood growth. As detailed elsewhere in this handbook for adults, a potential risk of chelator therapy in children is the apparently paradoxical worsening of neuropsychiatric symptoms following treatment initiation [28–32]. Bis-choline tetrathiomolybdate

(WTX101), a potent copper chelator that has not been linked to treatment-related neurological deterioration, is under development and, in the future, may provide a reliable therapeutic alternative. However, WTX101 remains an investigational agent and is currently unavailable for pediatric WD.

Zinc treatment is often the preferred treatment of very young and asymptomatic or presymptomatic children; as for adults, it is also a reasonable option for maintenance therapy. Pediatric dosing of zinc (particularly for the very young patient) is based on scarce age-specific data. In an initial study, zinc was effectively administered at 25 mg twice daily for patients 1–5 years old, 25 mg thrice daily for those 6–15 years old, and 50 mg thrice daily for older children (or those who weigh more than 125 pounds) [33]. Several other small studies generally confirm that these doses are safe and effective to treat WD in children based on clinical and biochemical parameters and basal urinary copper excretion [34–37]. As for adults, zinc is generally well tolerated, although gastric irritation can limit its use. Because this irritation typically occurs while fasting before breakfast with the first morning dose, consuming it midmorning is sometimes useful. Also, the salt used as zinc linker may be the culprit for the gastric complication. Hence, another way to potentially circumvent this problem is by consuming a different zinc preparation (e.g., changing from zinc acetate to sulfate to gluconate). However, there may be differences in absorption between the zinc salts, and it is important to monitor the patient for the effectiveness of the chosen preparation, that it is absorbed and achieving the same effect on keeping the patient clinically stable.

Untreated WD is fatal and medical treatment is lifelong. Prompt initiation of treatment following the diagnosis of WD in asymptomatic patients prevents the onset of hepatic and neurological complications of the disease [9, 10]. Interestingly, poor compliance with therapy is associated with the development of hepatic and neurological impairment in a considerable proportion of these presymptomatic patients identified through family screening [9]. These data highlight both the importance of early treatment and the difficulty with adherence in the asymptomatic population. The precise age to begin therapy in presymptomatic children is unknown. However, treatment is generally initiated at around 2–3 years old, because clinical manifestations of WD are rarely seen before this age [11]. Furthermore, the risk of treatment-related copper depletion during a critical stage of neurological development is a concern when treating very young asymptomatic patients (below 2–3 years of age), particularly since reliable monitoring of copper status is challenging.

Several aspects of WD therapy are especially challenging in young patients. A frequent problem with treatment is the need for multiple daily medication doses. This is especially an issue for zinc with three times daily dosing and the need for a midday dose in children attending school. Another frequent issue encountered is the need for some of these medications (D-penicillamine, trientine, and WTX101) to be kept cold, requiring careful forethought for storage (especially during activities away from the home). Because the bioavailability of chelators and zinc is decreased by foods, they need to be consumed at least 1 h before or 2 h after eating or drinking (anything but water), further complicating their consumption.

Young children or those with swallowing difficulties may struggle with consuming medication tablets as these need to be ingested whole without crushing. An effective method of teaching children to swallow tablets is by initially practicing with small-sized candies and gradually increasing their size until they become comfortable ingesting those of similar dimensions as the medication pills. Also, the use of special cups with pill holders may be useful in this regard. Trientine is exquisitely sensitive to moisture and is quickly degraded in water; thus, this medication cannot be compounded as a liquid. By contrast, D-penicillamine and zinc can be prepared as liquid solutions, but these formulations are typically more costly than their tablet counterparts and recently have not been available for purchase; additionally, compounding costs may not be covered by insurance. Also, because compounded formulations are not federally regulated, they are less likely to have been thoroughly tested for potency and contamination and may have different shelf lives than the capsule or tablet formulations. Finally, practitioners need to remain vigilant about the potential risks of overtreatment associated with copper depletion and deficiency when treating WD, particularly in very young children.

Treatment adherence is key in ensuring successful outcomes in the management of chronic illnesses. Medical compliance in infants, toddlers, and young children is exclusively determined by parents and caregivers. Providing these individuals with educational materials detailing the disease process, treatment rationale, and expectations is critically important in this process [36]. It is also essential to provide information about complications and common treatment-related side effects and offer practical ways to address these (e.g., adjusting a zinc dose to midmorning for gastric irritation). This is especially necessary with complex treatment regimens. Helping patients, caregivers, and families link medication schedules to regular activities and daily routines that create habits may also enhance compliance. Similarly, rewarding appropriate behavior and making adherence "fun" encourage compliance. For example, providing "stickers" or "stars" on a chart for ingesting medicines and rewarding upon the acquisition of a predefined number can enhance adherence, particularly in younger children. All involved in the care of children with WD should approach barriers with creative solutions, for example, as already mentioned, using gradually larger candies to teach young children to swallow pills. Also, finding a child-friendly laboratory for monitoring bloodwork may go a long way in alleviating anxiety that is typically associated with blood draws.

For parents and children, daily hassles of living, stress, and typical family conflict are some of the biggest barriers to compliance [38]. Addressing poor adherence requires the use of a comprehensive biopsychosocial and a team approach [39]. A therapeutic alliance involving close collaboration between child, parents, and clinician is important and should ideally be in place from the start of treatment. Involving the patient and parents in devising a plan to improve adherence is important.

References

1. Walsh JM. The liver in Wilson's disease (hepatolenticular degeneration). Diseases of the liver. Philadelphia: Lippincott; 1982. p. 1037–50.
2. Scheinberg IH, Sternlieb I. Wilson's disease. Philadelphia: WB Saunders; 1984.
3. SAK W. Progressive lenticular degeneration: a familial nervous disease associated with cirrhosis of the liver. Brain. 1912;34:295–507.
4. Iorio R, D'ambrosi M, Mazzarella G, et al. Early occurrence of hypertransaminasemia in a 13 month old child with Wilson disease. J Pediatr Gastroenterol Nutr. 2003;36:637–8.
5. Kim JW, Kim JH, Seo JK, et al. Genetically confirmed Wilson disease in a 9 month old boy with elevations of aminotransferases. World J Hepatol. 2013;5:156–9.
6. Abuduxikuer K, Li LT, Qiu YL, et al. Wilson disease with hepatic presentation in an eight month old boy. World J Gastroenterol. 2015;21:8981–4.
7. Sternlieb L, Scheinberg IH. Prevention of Wilsons disease in asymptomatic patients. N Engl J Med. 1968;2278:352–9.
8. Walsh JM. Diagnosis and treatment of presymptomatic Wilson's disease. Lancet. 1988;2(8608):435–7.
9. Dziezyc K, Karlinski M, Litwin T, et al. Compliant treatment with anti-copper agents prevents clinically overt Wilson's disease in presymptomatic patients. Eur J Neurol. 2014;21:332–7.
10. Dubbioso R, Ranucci G, Esposito M, et al. Subclinical neurological involvement does not develop if Wilson's disease is treated early. Parkinsonism Relat Disord. 2016 March;24:15–6.
11. Socha P, Janczyk W, Dhawan A, et al. Wilson's disease in children: a position paper by the Hepatology Committee of the European Society for paediatric gastroenterology, hepatology and nutrition. J Pediatr Gastroenterol Nutr. 2018;66:334–44.
12. Walsh JM. Cause of death in Wilson disease. Mov Disord. 2007;22:2216–20.
13. Scheinberg IH, Sterlieb I. Wilson disease and idiopathic copper toxicosis. Am J Clin Nutr. 1996;63:842S–5S.
14. O'Connor JA, Sokol RJ. Copper metabolism and copper storage disorders. In: Suchy FJ, Sokol RJ, Balistreri WF, editors. Liver disease in children. New York: Cambridge University Press; 2007. p. 626–60.

15. Wiernicka A, Dadalski M, janczyk W, et al. Early onset of Wilson disease: diagnostic challenges. J Pediatr Gastroenterol Nutr. 2017;65:555–60.
16. Cassin B, Soloman SAB. Dictionary of eye terminology. Third ed. Gainsville: Triad Publishing Company; 1997.
17. Roberts EA, Socha P. Wilson disease in children. Handbook of clinical neurology. Amsterdam: Elsevier; 2017. p. 145.
18. Martins Da Costa C, Baldwin D, Portmann B, et al. Value of urinary copper excretion after penicillamine challenge in the diagnosis of Wilson's disease. Hepatology. 1992;15:609–15.
19. Muller T, Koppikar S, Taylor RM, et al. Re-evaluation of the penicillamine challenge test in the diagnosis of Wilson's disease. In children. J Hepatol. 2007;47:270–6.
20. Schilsky ML. Non-invasive testing for Wilson disease: revisiting the d-penicillamine challenge test. J Hepatol. 2007;47(2):172–3.
21. Nicastro E, Ranucci G, Vajro P, et al. Re-evaluation of the diagnostic criteria for Wilson disease in children with mild liver disease. Hepatology. 2010;52:1948.
22. Roberts EA, Schilsky ML. Diagnosis and treatment of Wilson disease: an update. Hepatology. 2008;47:2089–111.
23. Dezsofi OA, Baumann U, Dhawan A, Durmaz O, Fischler B, Hadzic N, Hierro L, Lacaille F, McLin VA, Nobili V, Socha P, Vajro P, Knisely AS. Liver biopsy in children: position paper of the ESPGHAN Hepatology Committee. J Pediatr Gastroenterol Nutr. 2015;60:408–20.
24. Cohen MB, HH A-K, Lambers D, Heubi JE. Complications of percutaneous liver biopsy in children. Gastroenterology. 1992;102:629.
25. Ferenci P, Steindl-Munda P, Vogel W, et al. Diagnostic value of quantitative hepatic copper determination in patients with Wilson's disease. Clin Gastroenterol Hepatol. 2005;3:811–8.
26. Arnon R, Calderon JF, Schilsky M, et al. Wilson disease in children: serum aminotransferases and urinary copper on triethylene tetramine dihydrochloride (trientine) treatment. J Pediatr Gastroenterol Nutr. 2007;44:596–602.
27. Taylor RM, Chen Y, Dhawan A. Triethylene tetramine dihydrochloride (trientine) in children with Wilson disease: experience at King's College hospital and review of the literature. Eur J Pediatr. 2009;168:1061–8.
28. Weiss KH, Thurrik F, Gotthardt DN, et al. Efficacy and safety of oral chelators in treatment of patients with Wilson disease. Clin Gastroenterol Hepatol. 2013;21:599–606.

29. Litwin T, Dzlezyc K, Karlinski M, et al. Early neurological worsening in patients with Wilson's disease. J Neurol Sci. 2015;355:162–7.
30. Czlonkowska A, Litwin T, Karlinski M, et al. D-penicillamine versus zinc sulfate as first line therapy in Wilson's disease. Eur J Neurol. 2014;21:599–606.
31. Paul AC, Varkki S, Yohannan NB, et al. Neurologic deterioration in a child with Wilson's disease on penicillamine therapy. Indian J Gastroenterol. 2003;22:104–5.
32. Kalita J, Kumar V, Chandra S, et al. Worsening of Wilson disease following penicillamine therapy. Eur Neurol. 2014;71:126–31.
33. Brewer GJ, Dick RD, Johnson V. Treatment of Wilson's disease with zinc XVI: treatment during pediatric years. J Lab Clin Med. 2001;137:191–8.
34. Mizuochi T, Kimuar A, Shimizu N, et al. Zinc monotherapy from time of diagnosis for young pediatric patients with presymptomatic Wilson disease. J Pediatric Gastroenterol. 2011;53:365–7.
35. Marcellini M, Di Ciommo V, Callea F, et al. Treatment of Wilsons disease with zinc from the time of diagnosis in pediatric patients: a single-hospital, 10 year follow-up study. J Lab Clin Med. 2005;145:139–43.
36. Shimizu N, Fujiwara J, Ohnishi S, et al. Effects of long-term zinc treatment in Japanese patients with Wilson disease: efficacy, stability, and copper metabolism. Transl Res. 2010;156:350–7.
37. Eda K, Mizuochi T, Iwama I, et al. Zinc monotherapy for young children with presymptomatic Wilson disease: a multicenter study in Japan. J Gastroenterol Hepatol. 2018;33:264–9.
38. Dawood OT, Izham M, Ibrahim M, et al. Medication compliance among children. World J Pediatr. 2010;6:200–2.
39. Lask B. Motivating children and adolescents to improve adherence. Journal of Paediatrics. 2003;143:430–3.

Chapter 10
Wilson Disease: Special Circumstances

Michelle Camarata and Michael L. Schilsky

Presurgical and Peri-operative Management of the Patient with Wilson Disease

The consideration for surgical management of patients with Wilson disease should include considerations that are appropriate for any patient undergoing surgery, but also need to include

M. Camarata
Department of Gastroenterology and Hepatology, Royal Surrey County Hospital, Guildford, Surrey, UK

Department of Clinical and Experimental Medicine, University of Surrey, Guildford, Surrey, UK

Department of Surgery, Section of Transplant and Immunology, Yale School of Medicine, New Haven, CT, USA
e-mail: michelle.camarata@yale.edu

M. L. Schilsky (✉)
Division of Digestive Diseases and Transplant and Immunology, Departments of Medicine and Surgery, Yale University, New Haven, CT, USA
e-mail: michael.schilsky@yale.edu

M. L. Schilsky (ed.), *Management of Wilson Disease*, Clinical Gastroenterology, https://doi.org/10.1007/978-3-319-91527-2_10

consideration of how to adjust medication dosages for chelation and how to deal with dosages during times when nothing is allowed by mouth.

Patients with advanced liver disease must consider that there may be increased operative risk due to their liver disease. This typically occurs when the patient has cirrhosis and has decompensated disease (see section on liver disease, chapter 5). Avoidance of any elective procedures is recommended for these patients. However, in patients with stable cirrhosis without complications, surgery or other procedures may be considered. There should be attention to the platelet count and also the INR as a low platelet count (typically below 50,000) and elevated INR (above 1.5) may indicate a higher risk for postoperative bleeding. For some high-risk procedures, patients may need a transfusion of platelets (or use of a platelet stimulating factor) and plasma to prevent bleeding.

Another consideration for operations and procedures is wound healing. Copper plays an important role in cross-linking collagen by virtue of it being a cofactor for lysyl oxidase. For patients on zinc with good copper balance, there is no dose modification recommended. For those on chelation with D-penicillamine or trientine, a dose reduction of ~50% is recommended to begin about a week prior to the procedure and continue until there is adequate wound healing.

There are times when patients cannot take medication or food perioperatively. If the time period is only for a few days, then treatment likely can be temporarily held and resumed when possible given that copper intake is also likely low during this time. If there are prolonged periods of perioperative fasting when patients need to receive food supplements from an enteral or gastric feeding tube, then liquid preparations of dissolved drug or zinc given separate from food can be considered.

Treatment in Pregnancy for Wilson Disease

In considering treatment of WD during pregnancy, both the health of the fetus and the mother must be considered. For the mother, it is essential that treatment for WD continues during pregnancy to avoid complications from WD such as worsening liver disease or development of neurologic symptoms. For the fetus, it is very important to pick therapies with the lowest risk for fetal complications while enhancing fetal growth and development.

When patients are on zinc therapy, there is no dose reduction needed when patients are trying to conceive or during the pregnancy if the patient is well treated and has stable liver function and stable or no neurologic disease. If the patient or physician is concerned about keeping a patient on chelation therapy during pregnancy, then switching to zinc ahead of pregnancy is an option. However, switching during pregnancy may not be the best course of action as patients may not tolerate the zinc due to worsening issues of reflux and dyspepsia due to uterine enlargement and increased intra-abdominal pressure from the developing fetus and amniotic fluid.

If patients are on chelation therapy, their current regimen might be maintained as a recent series showed successful pregnancies under all available medical therapies [1]. However, with respect to best practices, dosing modifications are suggested for those with stable disease on chelation therapy as early as possible because the risk to the fetus for any teratogenicity is highest in the first trimester of life and risk of fetal copper deficiency would be lowered [2]. Therefore, exposure to either D-penicillamine or trientine should be minimized by dose reduction as early as possible during the pregnancy or even in anticipation of the pregnancy. This means that female patients who are trying to become pregnant should consult their physician and consider minimizing treatment. If the dosage is reduced, the patient needs to step up monitoring frequency while on this lower dosage. What the safest dosage is for reduction of treatment is unknown, but on average, a 30–50% dose reduction with monitoring every 3–4 months is advised. Similarly, this would translate into monitoring once each trimester for pregnant patients. Once the patient delivers, then if there was no operative intervention, the medication can be returned to the prepregnancy dosage. If the delivery was by caesarian section or if an episiotomy was performed, then the therapy should remain at the lower dosage until there is wound healing.

The Earliest Age for Initiating Wilson Disease Therapy

One of the most difficult questions to answer when a new diagnosis of WD is made in neonates and very young children under the age of 3–4 years is when to initiate treatment. Most current recommendations are to wait until the age of 3–5 years as there are only rare reports of symptomatic disease before then. Furthermore, the neonatal and early growth periods are important for neuronal development, and copper is a necessary element during this time.

Arguments for earlier initiation of treatment are that one can prevent any development of hepatic copper toxicity by reducing the concentration of copper that is already elevated in the newborn liver. In a report by Socio et al. [3], two asymptomatic patients began early treatment with D-penicillamine at ages 2 and 3 years. However, data from these patients showed that they had a low non-ceruloplasmin copper at baseline, and it is possible that they may have done just as well or better if treatment were delayed and the only intervention was a low copper diet. If treatment is initiated in the very young, monitoring should include both growth and development as well as laboratory monitoring for copper deficiency such as blood counts looking for anemia, neutropenia, or thrombocytopenia. Other issues regarding which medication to choose in the very young and how to administer the medication in young patients are not well described. Issues regarding giving medication to pediatric patients are discussed in chapter 9.

Breastfeeding While on Wilson Disease Therapy

The evidence base on whether it is safe to breastfeed while on treatment for Wilson disease is limited, and currently no randomized controlled trials have been performed. Currently, guidelines do not support breastfeeding on treatment although there are reports of infants that have not had adverse effects while doing so.

Limited information indicates that both trientine and penicillamine are not detectable in breast milk. In a small study of four patients receiving trientine for WD at dosages of 1000, 1500, and 1750 mg, trientine was not detectable by HPLC in the breast milk of any of the maternal milk samples [5]. Four patients received penicillamine for WD at dosages of 800, 600, and 500 mg daily while breastfeeding, and it also was not detectable by HPLC in the breast milk of any of the maternal milk samples [5]. In infants who breastfeed infrequently, taking the medication straight after breastfeeding and avoiding breastfeeding for 4–6 h should further minimize the amount of drug in breast milk.

Zinc and copper serum levels have been shown to be normal in a study of three infants breastfed on maternal treatment of WD with trientine [6]. Data on milk concentrations of zinc and copper in patients on treatment with trientine is conflicting one abstract reporting normal breast milk concentrations [4], while another by the same authors reported lower concentrations [5]. In patients breastfeeding on treatment with penicillamine for WD, the levels of zinc and copper in breast milk have been shown to be reduced [5–8].

Data demonstrating the effect of treatment with chelation therapy on breastfed infants is limited. A case report of one woman who had breastfed two infants on treatment with penicillamine 750 mg daily reported prolonged icterus in one infant which was felt to be unlikely related to penicillamine [9]. Another woman taking penicillamine 1500 mg daily for a different disorder, cystinuria, breastfed her infant for 3 months with no apparent side effects in her infant [10]. A center in Turkey reported on 23 infants that were breastfed by mothers with WD on treatment over a 20-year period. Although all infants were breastfed, the extent and duration were not specified. Drug doses were reduced during pregnancy. Twenty-one mothers were on treatment with penicillamine 600 mg and zinc 100 mg daily, one was treated with trientine 600 mg and zinc 100 mg, and one was treated with zinc monotherapy once a day. One premature infant died at 3 weeks of age (maternal drug not specified). No other infant complications occurred over a median of 51 months of follow-up (range 13–105 months) [11].

Safety of zinc treatment during lactation has not been clearly established. Elemental zinc is known to be excreted in breast milk [12]. The recommended daily allowance of elemental zinc during lactation is 19 mg during the first 6 months and 16 mg during the second 6 months. Zinc is required for normal growth and development in infants that are breastfed. The effect of breastfed infants at higher dosages used in WD is not known. The concern is that maternal treatment with zinc while breastfeeding may lead to copper deficiency in the nursing infant.

Currently, due to lack of supporting evidence, breastfeeding under chelation therapy and on zinc treatment is not recommended although there are reports that have demonstrated no adverse effects on infants while breastfeeding on treatment with chelators and zinc [2, 9–11, 13].

In summary, medication adjustments for patients undergoing surgery and during pregnancy are recommended for those on chelation therapy. Breastfeeding is currently not recommended in patients on treatment for WD. When to start therapy in young patients and which is the best therapy will need further study to delineate best practice recommendations.

Bibliography

1. Pfeiffenberger J, Mogler C, Gotthardt DN, et al. Hepatobiliary malignancies in Wilson disease. Liver Int. 2015;35(5):1257–66.
2. Roberts EA, Schilsky ML. Diagnosis and treatment of Wilson disease: an update. Hepatology. 2008;47:2089–111.
3. Izumi Y. Can mothers with Wilson's disease give breast milk to their infant? Teikyo Med J. 2012;35:17–24.
4. Shiga K, Kaga H, Kodama H, et al. Copper and zinc concentrations in the breast milk of mothers with Wilson disease and effects on infants. J Inherit Metab Dis. 2006;29:139. https://doi.org/10.1007/s10545-006-9995-6.

5. Byron MA. Treatment of rheumatic diseases. Br Med J. 1987;294:336–8.
6. Ramsey-Goldman R, Schilling E. Optimum use of disease-modifying and immunosuppressive antirheumatic agents during pregnancy and lactation. Clin Immunother. 1996;5:40–58.
7. Messner U, Gunter HH, Niesert S. Wilson disease and pregnancy. Review of the literature and case report. Z Geburtshilfe Neonatol. 1998;202:77–9.
8. Gregory MC, Mansell MA. Pregnancy and cystinuria. Lancet. 1983;2:1158–60.
9. Demir K, Soyer OM, Karaca C, et al. The course of pregnancy in Wilson's disease-once center, 20 year experience. Gastroenterology. 2014;146 S-1009. Abstract TU1834.
10. Krebs NF, Reidinger CJ, Hartley S, et al. Zinc supplementation during lactation: effects on maternal status and milk zinc concentrations. Am J Clin Nutr. 1995;61:1030–6.
11. Ferenci P, Czonkowska A, Stremmel W, et al. EASL clinical practice guidelines: Wilson's disease. J Hepatol. 2012;56:671–85.
12. Sócio SA, Ferreira AR, Fagundes EDT, et al. Doença de Wilson em crianças e adolescentes: diagnóstico e tratamento (Wilson's disease in children and adolescents: diagnosis and treatment). Rev paul pediatr. 2010;28(2):134–40.
13. Kaga F, Kodama H, Siga K, et al. Copper and zinc status in the breast milk of mothers with Wilson disease. J Inherit Metab Dis. 2008;31:157.

Chapter 11
Liver Transplantation for Wilson Disease

Tamir Miloh and Michael L. Schilsky

Introduction

The natural history of untreated Wilson disease (WD) is progressive liver failure and/or neurological deterioration which leads to death. Liver transplantation (LT) for WD allows for replacement of the defective or absent ATP7B copper transporter responsible for WD, which is mainly expressed in the primary liver cells (hepatocytes) in the liver. Approximately 5% of WD patients present with acute liver

T. Miloh
Pediatric Hepatology and Liver Transplant Medicine, Texas Children's Hospital, Houston, TX, USA

Baylor College of Medicine, Houston, TX, USA
e-mail: tamiloh@texaschildrens.org

M. L. Schilsky (✉)
Division of Digestive Diseases and Transplant and Immunology, Departments of Medicine and Surgery, Yale University, New Haven, CT, USA
e-mail: michael.schilsky@yale.edu

M. L. Schilsky (ed.), *Management of Wilson Disease*, Clinical Gastroenterology, https://doi.org/10.1007/978-3-319-91527-2_11

failure (ALF) which rarely responds to medical management and requires urgent evaluation and listing for LT with the highest priority for transplant, status 1a as designated by the United Network for Organ Sharing (UNOS). Approximately 10% of WD patients present with advanced end-stage liver disease (ESLD) and either fail or are not responsive to medical therapy and therefore require a LT [1]. Options for donor organs included deceased donors (cadaveric) and orthotopic (replacement of the recipient's liver), living liver donation where a partial liver is implanted in place of the recipient's liver. In addition, though rarely performed, there is an option to augment liver function by placing a partial or whole liver into the patient in addition to the patient's own liver, and this is known as heterotopic or auxiliary LT. Data from the USA and other countries demonstrate excellent short-term and long-term outcomes for LT for WD [2, 3]. LT is recommended for WD-related liver disease, whereas LT for severe neurologic disease remains controversial.

Indications for Liver Transplantation

Acute Liver Failure (ALF)

Approximately 5% of patients of patients with ALF have WD [4]. ALF is the primary presentation for approximately 5% of WD patients, occurring more frequently in females (4:1) and in the second decade of life [5]. ALF due to WD may also develop in some patients with previously well-treated liver disease following discontinuation of their medical therapy [6]. Acute liver failure (ALF) is defined as acute onset of coagulopathy (INR > 2) and hepatic encephalopathy in a patient without known pre-existing liver disease and with an illness of <26-week duration. The injury to liver cells caused by copper in ALF due to WD involves different mechanisms known as apoptosis and acute cellular necrosis [7]. Patients may have nonimmune hemolytic anemia and renal dysfunction as a consequence of the release of large amounts of copper from injured liver cells. Early identification of patients with ALF due to WD is critical as these patients rarely respond to medical management and are at high risk of mortality without a LT.

Patients presenting with ALF due to WD should be referred promptly to a liver transplant center, rapidly evaluated, and listed for LT. While on the transplant wait list, the therapeutic goal is to rapidly reduce the excess circulating copper released from injured liver cells to reduce red blood cell loss by hemolysis, spare the kidney from further injury from copper complexes that cause renal tubular injury, and slow further injury to the remaining functioning liver cells prior to LT. Strategies that have been used to rapidly lower copper from the circulation include plasma exchange [8], albumin dialysis [9], plasmapheresis [10], hemofiltration [11], fractioned plasma separation and absorption (FPSA) [12], liver dialysis with single-pass albumin dialysis (SPAD) [13], and early institution of renal replacement therapy and molecular adsorbent recirculating system (MARS) [14]. The choice of a particular therapy may depend on the availability of the devices needed to perform these treatments and the experience of the treating team with their use. These strategies may also improve patient outcomes after LT as some of the injury to other organs that is caused by copper during this critical time can be mitigated. Patients with ALF due to WD should be referred to a liver transplant center, where they should be evaluated promptly and barring any factors that would prevent a good outcome, listed as status 1a (see organ allocation policy below).

LT for Chronic Liver Disease

Patients with ESLD due to WD typically present in the third decade of life and are usually older than patients presenting with ALF. Patients may have ESLD at the time of initial WD diagnosis In some that are treated, the disease may progress over time, mostly due to nonadherence with medical therapy for WD or injury from other unrelated liver disease. LT is indicated for patients with WD and chronic liver disease who develop severe hepatic insufficiency and decompensated cirrhosis, defined as having jaundice, ascites, variceal bleeding, or hepatorenal syndrome. Patients with ESLD who do not fulfill criteria for ALF are listed with their PELD/MELD score with appropriate sodium adjustment. In some cases, an appeal for exception is required (see organ allocation below).

In some of these patients, chelation therapy may be effective and thereby avoid LT [15]. The AASLD guidelines on WD suggest that a 3-month trial of medical therapy be considered; however, if there is a decline in the clinical or biochemical status, patients should be evaluated for LT earlier [5, 16]. The Nazer score was initially proposed to help determine if medical therapy is useful [8]. This has been updated to the modified WD scoring system [9]. This scoring system that uses biochemical data and data from blood counts can be applied to predict the response to medical therapy, with scores >11 predicting death without LT [17]. However, there have been cases reported of successful chelation therapy without LT of WD patients with scores above 10 [18], and therefore, the trajectory of the patients score must be taken into consideration. Overall, it is recommended that patients with advanced disease are evaluated for LT and given a trial of medical therapy while on the LT wait list. Continuous and sustained clinical and biochemical improvement that correlates with a decrease in their modified WD score would then warrant reassessment of the patient's need for LT. Some patients may even be made inactive or taken off the LT wait list if their condition remains improved.

The decision to evaluate, list, and transplant patients with WD may be different among transplant centers. In a retrospective review of LT at multiple centers in the USA and Europe, data from 55 transplants where 43 survived over a span of 20 years showed some transplanted with scores below the threshold noted by Nazer et al. [8], perhaps reflecting center choice more than objective evidence that treatment had failed [19]. Other factors such as continued GI bleeding from esophageal or gastric varices or the presence of ascites or hepatic encephalopathy independent of the overall liver score may have driven the choices to move forward with LT at that time.

While on the LT wait list, patients should be managed for any complications that can arise from their chronic liver disease including management of complications of portal hypertension, screening and surveillance for esophageal and gastric varices, screening and surveillance for hepatocellular carcinoma, other complications of portal hypertension affecting oxygenation due to blood shunting in the lungs (hepatopulmonary syndrome) or changes due to increased pressures in the lung arterial circulation (portopulmonary hypertension), management of volume with sodium restriction and diuretics, treatment for hepatic encephalopathy, and treatment and prophylaxis for spontaneous bacterial peritonitis. In addition, optimization of nutrition is important to avoid malnourishment and loss of muscle mass (sarcopenia) that typically can worsen as a patient's liver disease progresses. For future transplantation, this is important to help with post-LT recovery.

LT for Neuropsychiatric Manifestations of WD

LT primarily for neurologic and psychiatric manifestations of WD without the presence of acute or chronic liver failure is controversial for two main reasons. Patients with neurologic disease may improve with chelation therapy. There are no firm clinical or radiologic criteria to accurately predict neurologic outcomes for treatment of WD patients with neurologic impairment. LT carries significant morbidity and mortality risk and requires lifelong immunosuppressive medications. However, restoration of normal biliary copper excretion with LT will over time reduce brain copper accumulation and prevent further injury. There are some reports of improvement in neurologic symptoms after LT [20–23]. Overall in 56–77% of the cases with neurologic symptoms due to WD at the time of LT, complete recovery is possible, usually at least 6 months after LT, and may take up to 18 months [15, 21, 23]. However, there are other studies noting permanent disability, severe injury and worsening of symptoms and quality of life, and even death post-LT for WD patients with neurologic features pretransplant [3, 15, 24–28]. Patients transplanted solely for neurologic WD had a worse prognosis than patients transplanted for liver disease alone [3]. In this study from France, three of the seven patients transplanted for neurologic WD that had severe axial Parkinson's syndrome died from infection at 2, 4, and 36 months post-LT without any neurologic improvement. The other patients with severe intractable neurologic impairment required continuous nursing care prior to LT. Neurologic dysfunction could increase the potential risk of infection, either through a prolonged duration of being bedridden, frequent hospitalization, or also the risk of aspiration. However, these same authors report that one patient with dystonia and chorea, another with dystonia and myoclonia, and a third with ataxia and frontal syndrome were reported to have had major improvements. The other 19 patients transplanted for hepatic indications had mixed neurologic post-LT outcomes; 3 recovered, 5 partially recovered, 1 was unchanged, and 1 worsened after LT.

It is recommended that WD patients with neurologic abnormalities be evaluated by a neurologist, preferably a movement disorder specialist, before transplantation. It may be helpful to use a validated neurologic rating scale to assess patients' degree of neurologic involvement before and after transplant, especially if neurologic symptoms are present. The Unified Wilson Disease Rating Scale (UWDRS) for neurologic and psychiatric features of WD has been used for this purpose and was applied before and after LT in a study performed in Turkey, indicating demonstrating improvement after LT [29].

There are no good reports of outcomes for psychiatric symptoms post-LT in WD. Without standardization of the examination of patients before and after LT, it is difficult to evaluate psychiatric outcome, especially given the potential for many of the posttransplant medications and hospitalization to influence a patient's symptoms.

The presence of psychiatric symptoms could be considered as a partial contraindication for LT if they are severe and there are concerns regarding such issues as suicidality and adherence to the use of the required medications that would follow LT. Patients with a combination of neuropsychiatric conditions deserve careful evaluation. LT may also be contraindicated in cases of severe neurologic impairment where there may be little chance for improvement. This is sometimes very challenging to determine given the lack of good information about predictability of recovery; however, a useful rule of thumb is that the longer symptoms have been present, the lower likelihood there is of their recovery.

Despite confidence in our ability to determine which patients with liver disease are doing poorly with medical therapy and are in need of LT, it is still unclear when and whether LT should be considered in patients with neuropsychiatric manifestations of WD not responding to medical therapy. For instance, important questions of how long to treat before declaring a treatment failure and which treatment at what dosage to use remain to a large degree unanswered. The term "non-response" therefore requires better definition in this population, and better studies are needed to guide future care. Overall, the decision to perform LT in WD patients solely on the basis of their neurologic impairment should still be considered experimental, and data carefully collected to inform future use of LT for these individuals.

Organ Allocation Policy for LT and WD

Patients older than 12 years of age are placed on the national UNOS wait list and prioritized according to the model for end-stage liver disease (MELD) scoring system. The MELD score is calculated using variables that are determined by blood testing. These variables are the INR, creatinine, and bilirubin levels, with a more recent attribution of extra points to those with low serum sodium (hyponatremia) (MELDNa). Organs are offered to candidates on the wait list in accordance with their degree of illness. The sickest patients as determined by their MELDNa score are offered organs first, with consideration for the appropriate blood type match. In addition, the size of the organ may matter, and there is some size matching between donor and potential recipient that has to be determined by the surgeons who are performing the operation. For instance, an extremely large organ from a donor may need to be either split for use or declined for a smaller recipient due to practical size considerations for the transplant operation.

Patients younger than 12 years are prioritized on the UNOS wait list according to the pediatric end-stage liver disease (PELD) score that differs slightly from MELD in that it additionally uses the patients' serum albumin and age and whether they have "failure to thrive," a term referring to a lack of appropriate normal growth and development. If the calculated score does not reflect disease severity, there is a process of appealing for exception points to increase a patient's priority on the waiting list. An appeal can be made to the UNOS regional review board, and a group of transplant physicians on the board have to approve the application to increase points on the wait list. Patients presenting with acute liver failure (INR > 2 and encephalopathy) can be listed differently as status 1a, granting top priority on the LT wait list. Therefore, confirming a diagnosis of WD is important, so that patients with ALF due to WD with advanced fibrosis or cirrhosis (which would otherwise disqualify these patients for this designation) may achieve the highest priority for organ allocation. Policies for organ allocation can be found at http://optn.transplant.hrsa.gov/media/1200/optn_policies.pdf#nameddest=Policy_09.

The Eurotransplant, which is the European counterpart to UNOS, gives a priority to WD patients presenting with ALF as well. Their policy can be found at http://www.eurotransplant.org/cms/index.php?page=public_meld.

UNOS policy for organ allocation also allows increased priority for transplantation of patients with liver disease with hepatocellular carcinoma (HCC) that meet special criteria.

The HCC must be what is known as Milan criteria (three tumors less than 3 cm or one less than 5 cm) and confined to the liver without vascular invasion (as seen on imaging) and must not be able to be surgically resected due to location or to underlying liver disease. Recent UNOS policy changes also permit slightly larger HCC with total size of less than 8 cm in aggregate to be treated, and if the remaining tumor is within Milan criteria, candidates may also be granted increased priority. A meta-analysis showed a lower overall annual risk of 0.04% (95% CI 0.01–0.10) of the development of HCC in WD patients, a lower rate compared with patients with cirrhosis of other etiologies [30]. However, further prospective study is needed to know the true incidence of development of HCC in WD patients.

Options for LT for WD

Orthotopic LT for WD

The liver has two lobes (right and left) and eight lobules (1–8). Donor livers that are utilized for transplantation may be whole livers or part of the liver, segmental grafts. The technical variants may be reduced size or split livers that can be used for LT. Here usually the smaller left lateral segment (liver segments 2 + 3) is used for children, and the extended right lobe is used for adult recipients. Overall the success rate using split and whole livers is equivalent [31]. Cadaveric or deceased liver donors may originate from brain death (DBD) or non-heart beating or cardiac death (DCD). Some donors may be considered as increased risk, for example, due to their incarceration, drug use, history of hepatitis B or C, or other medical issues such as infection or cancer. In these settings, the potential recipient is made aware of the donor risk factors and asked to either consent to use the organ or decline its use for them. The benefit of using an increased risk donor should be considered against the cost of not doing the transplant in the recipient, i.e., risk of dying waiting for an organ while on the waiting list. There is a shortage of donor organ availability, and there is approximately 20% mortality on the transplant wait list. While accepting a higher-risk organ is a way to potentially reduce time on the wait list, another way is to perform living donor LT. Living donor liver transplant, where a part of a liver from a donor is given to the recipient, can be used successfully for patients with WD, even when the parent is a carrier (heterozygous) for WD [32]. In living donor LT, the partial liver remaining in the donor and the partial graft given to the recipient grow in size to match their appropriate individual liver size (i.e., proportional to their own size). Before considering living donor LT, patients have to first be suitable candidates for LT and then placed on the UNOS wait list. Living liver donation offers the option for a scheduled LT at a time that is best for both recipient and donor. The living donor is assessed thoroughly by a separate dedicated medical team to assure the suitability and safety of the living liver donation.

Auxiliary or Heterotopic LT for WD

Auxiliary liver grafts are partial grafts that are placed in the patient in addition to some or all of the patient's original liver. For WD, the ability to clear copper from the circulation to bile is enhanced by the auxiliary liver. Later on, if there is adequate recovery of the native liver, it is possible to withdraw immune suppression, leaving the auxiliary graft to undergo acute and chronic rejection. In a case report on auxiliary LT for a patient with WD, Park et al. reaffirm the great degree of technical demand and the potential problems, such as the development of HCC that are associated with leaving an injured organ in place, limiting the use of this technology [33].

Another case of auxiliary liver transplant was performed on a 36-year-old with WD without cirrhosis but with neurologic symptoms. The patient was treated with chelation therapy and had normal liver enzymes. The donor was the patient's 57-year-old father. The operation was performed utilizing the left lobe, and the graft-to-recipient weight ratio was excellent for safety and function at 1%. The patient's serum ceruloplasmin normalized after the transplant and their neurologic symptoms improved. Liver function tests were normal. These authors concluded that progressive neurological deterioration with no hepatic insufficiency may be considered a suitable indication for auxiliary partial orthotopic liver transplant [34]. However, it is unclear whether use of alternative medical therapies or a longer period of treatment with the same therapy might have yielded a different outcome with therapy and perhaps transplantation avoided in this patient.

Living Donor Liver Transplant (LDLT) for Wilson Disease

The worldwide shortage of donor livers led to LDLT as an alternative to the conventional deceased donor LT (orthotopic liver transplantation and heterotopic auxiliary liver transplantation). LDLT is essential for pediatric patients who require reduced size grafts, in some countries where deceased donor (cadaveric) transplantation is not culturally or religiously accepted or allowed, and for individuals in need of LT but who are not prioritized by the current allocation system. When considering live donation, surgical risks to the donor as well as disease transmission and other complications that may affect the liver recipient's outcome are assessed prior to LT. As most living donors are related to patients, usually parents, children, or siblings, for LDLT for WD, it is important to exclude those donors who may either be WD patients themselves or who might have other conditions jeopardizing their own or the recipient outcome. These assurances are obtained by careful clinical and biochemical testing that sometimes includes the analysis of a liver biopsy from the donor for histology and liver copper content. Molecular diagnostic testing for *ATP7B* mutations now also contributes to potential donor selection. Before acceptance as a candidate for donation for LDLT, a person's age, evidence for any clinical feature of liver disease, and recipient indication for transplantation, time on the waiting list, outcome of medical treatment, other extrahepatic conditions (especially neurologic status in WD), and serological data are all important considerations in determining need and timing of LT.

In addition to excluding that a potential liver donor was not actually a patient with WD, it was initially unknown whether those relatives who were carriers for WD would provide the same excellent outcomes as unaffected donors. Data on LDLT for WD by several centers demonstrate that the use of a living related donor who is a heterozygote carrier for WD is safe and provides effective function in the recipient with WD [35].

There are reports that long-term graft survival is increased and rejection rates decreased in patients undergoing LDLT. This may be explained by multiple factors including immunologic advantages, improved donor quality and shortened cold ischemia, and psychosocial factors leading to increased adherence [36].

Outcomes and Monitoring After LT

Since the first successful LT for WD in 1963, WD with liver failure has been considered an appropriate indication for LT with the ability to achieve excellent long-term survival. This has been supported by a number of publications summarized in Table 11.1. Copper metabolism normalizes with a restoration of activity of the ATP7B copper transporter in liver cells, helping to reduce extrahepatic copper overload over time. Early after LT, there may be a surge in urinary copper excretion due to the excess accumulation of copper outside of the liver. Over an average period of 6 months, there is normalization of the urine copper excretion in most post-LT patients as serum ceruloplasmin, serum copper concentration, and urinary copper excretion return to normal. Portal hypertensive symptoms will improve after transplanting a cirrhotic liver.

TABLE 11.1 Outcomes of patients with Wilson disease who underwent liver transplantation

							Patient survival		
OLT	LD	ALF	ESLD	Neuro only	Pediatrics	Adults	1-year	5-year	Country and reference
	1 auxiliary			1		1			Turkey: Haberal (2017)
107		21	86				86%	82%	Iran: Lankarani (2016)
136	4	64	57		45	75	89%	87%	France: Gulliaud (2014)
30		11	18	1					Austria: Beinhardt (2014)
19		8	11				78%	65%	Germany: Weiss (2013)
	36	2	34		10	26	92%	75%	China: Cheng (2009)
	32	21	11		24	8	91%	84%	Japan: Yoshitoshi (2009)
37		8	29				89%	76%	Italy: Medici (2005)
165	5	103	67		51	119	92%	90%	USA: Arnon (2001)
17		11	6		3	14	87%		USA: Emre (2001)
55		21	32	1			79%		USA/Europe: Schilsky (1994)

Shown are results from studies for patients who had orthotopic liver transplantation (OLT), living donor transplant (LD). Indications for transplant were acute liver failure (ALF), end-stage liver disease (ESLD), or neurologic symptoms (Neuro) for adult and pediatric patients

Neurologic symptoms may improve, stabilize, or worsen after LT. Psychiatric symptoms usually do not improve after LT, but this has not been as rigorously evaluated.

Several reports support the excellent short- and long-term outcomes for post-LT pediatric and adult patients transplanted for ALF or ESLD due to WD. The results improved in more recent years due to improvements in surgical technique and medical management (LT post-2000 have better patient outcomes). In a UNOS registry study that included data collected by the US transplant registry for 170 pediatric patients and 400 adults with WD, graft and patient 1-year survival was 90.1% and 89% and 88% and 96%, respectively, superior to many other LT indications [2]. Analysis of a comparable European transplant registry reported no statistically significant difference in patient survival rates according to gender, age at transplantation, blood group, CHILD-Pugh score, and medical therapy or whether LT was performed for ALF or for ESLD due to WD [37]. The major cause of post-surgical death was sepsis. Data from France showed excellent overall patient long-term survival rates post-LT for WD of 89% at 1 year and 87% at 5, 10, 15, and 20 years [3]. The major cause of mortality after LT was sepsis, but some also died from intracranial hypertension due to brain swelling, bleeding, cardiogenic shock, ARDS, and hyperacute graft rejection and for unknown reasons.

The excellent long-term outcomes post-LT for WD may be explained by the fact that in contrary to other indications for LT (HCV, NAFLD, HCC), WD does not recur in the graft. Also, with the relatively short period that elapsed between onset of the severe disease and LT in those with ALF, patients were not as debilitated as those with chronic ESLD. Patients with WD were transplanted at a relatively younger age and have a lower rate of other medical problems compared to other LT indications. Long-term renal function of WD patients after LT was excellent despite the high frequency of pre-liver copper-induced kidney injury, and patients who require pre-LT renal support (dialysis or equivalent) can be weaned off [25]. Following LT, there can be prolongation of kidney dysfunction from exposure to calcineurin inhibitors such as tacrolimus and cyclosporine A used for immune suppression following LT.

LDLT provides the same excellent results for LT for WD as deceased donor LT. In a large series, patient survival data at 1 and 5 years after LDLT was 91.7% and 75%, and corresponding graft survival was 86.1% and 75%, respectively [38]. Similarly a second series provided data of 1-, 5-, and 10-year cumulative patient survival rates of 90.6%, 83.7%, and 80%, respectively, following LDLT [39].

Immunosuppression After Liver Transplantation in WD Patients

Patients undergoing LT need to take lifelong immunosuppressant (IS) medication to prevent graft rejection. There is a very small subset that may develop tolerance and weaned off IS, and this is discussed below. Common IS agents used are tacrolimus, steroids, mycophenolate, azathioprine, and sirolimus. Each IS carries a unique spectrum of potential side effects. Dosing of tacrolimus, cyclosporine, everolimus, and sirolimus is managed by measurement of levels in the circulation. The trough levels (the lowest level in thc body prior to the next dose of medication) can be evaluated from serum and the dosage adjusted accordingly. The target level of IS post-LT changes with time from the transplant. In the early phase (usually the first 3 months), the target levels are higher and gradually decrease over time as the risk of rejection of the donor organ is highest in this time period. After the first 3–6 months, levels of these drugs are usually lower. However, in some patients with a history of graft rejection, higher levels need to be maintained, or a combination of IS agents is used in order to treat and prevent future rejection. There is a fine balance between adverse side effects of IS and benefit of preventing rejection of the donor organ. Young patients with ALF WD may have a functional immune system and require higher IS. However, the choice of IS and target levels may need to be customized for those with severe hepatic encephalopathy or neurologic injury prior to LT. Tacrolimus, the most common IS used after LT, can induce neurologic disease such as tremor, seizure, and PRESS. Therefore some advocate the use of cyclosporine A instead of tacrolimus as there theoretically may be less neurologic toxicity early on or alternatively consider medications such as everolimus or sirolimus after 8 weeks post-LT. To minimize neurologic complications, levels of tacrolimus or cyclosporine A may be kept at the low end of the therapeutic range (sometimes aided by using mycophenolate or azathioprine at the same time), and magnesium levels should be monitored and supplementation given to keep magnesium levels normal and the seizure threshold higher.. Patients with WD and renal disease may require IS regimens that are less nephrotoxic, such as keeping target levels of tacrolimus or cyclosporine A lower with the addition of mycophenolate or azathioprine. There are a few regimens for IS that avoid use of tacrolimus and cyclosporine as well for patients with advanced renal disease, but the risk of graft rejection may be higher, and there may be other complications with their use. However, in most patients with WD, renal function due to the copper load returns to normal after LT. Nephrotoxicity may develop over time due to the IS effect [40], and kidney function must be monitored closely.

Some pediatric and very rare adult patients are able to wean and ultimately withdraw dependency on immunosuppressant medication post-LT, including some with WD; however, protocols for withdrawal of these agents are still experimental [37]. Factors such as age (more favorable in pediatric patients) and time out from transplantation in addition to biochemical indices, gender, and rejection episodes contribute toward assessing the possibility of successful weaning. Further research on immunosuppressive medications and the basic mechanisms of transplant immunology will help improve long-term patient survival post-LT for all patients and thereby benefit those with WD who had LT.

Conclusion: The Future of LT for WD

Although medical therapies are available for WD, there is a role for LT for some patients with WD found either with ALF or with chronic ESLD beyond our capacity to restore function with medical therapy. LT for patients with neurologic WD without liver failure should be undertaken with caution and preferably as part of a research study to help guide its future use. Careful choices and monitoring of medications posttransplant can reduce the risk of seizure and allow better renal recovery in those with copper-induced acute kidney injury that occurred during their liver failure. Outcomes for LT for WD are excellent. LDLT helps expand the pool of livers for those in need of LT and allows for the optimal timing of transplantation to achieve best outcomes. Future advances in liver support devices in addition to novel methods for acutely lowering circulating copper may be useful for those with ALF due to WD and may someday bridge them to recovery instead of LT.

In summary, LT remains lifesaving for those with WD in need and restores normal copper metabolism by providing correction of the underlying metabolic defect present in the native liver of the recipient. In addition, for those transplanted for ESLD due to WD, portal hypertension and its complications are removed. Though gene therapy and even gene repair hold promise as future WD therapies, until we can universally detect this disorder in presymptomatic patients, there likely will continue to be a need for LT for WD in the future.

References

1. Schilsky ML. Liver transplantation for Wilson's disease. Ann N Y Acad Sci. 2014;1315:45–9.
2. Arnon R, et al. Liver transplantation for children with Wilson disease: comparison of outcomes between children and adults. Clin Transpl. 2011;25(1):E52–60.
3. Guillaud O, et al. Long term results of liver transplantation for Wilson's disease: experience in France. J Hepatol. 2014;60(3):579–89.

4. Ostapowicz G, et al. Results of a prospective study of acute liver failure at 17 tertiary care centers in the United States. Ann Intern Med. 2002;137(12):947–54.
5. Roberts EA, Schilsky ML, D. American Association for Study of Liver. Diagnosis and treatment of Wilson disease: an update. Hepatology. 2008;47(6):2089–111.
6. Walshe JM, Dixon AK. Dangers of non-compliance in Wilson's disease. Lancet. 1986;1(8485):845–7.
7. Strand S, et al. Hepatic failure and liver cell damage in acute Wilson's disease involve CD95 (APO-1/Fas) mediated apoptosis. Nat Med. 1998;4(5):588–93.
8. Kiss JE, Berman D, Van Thiel D. Effective removal of copper by plasma exchange in fulminant Wilson's disease. Transfusion. 1998;38(4):327–31.
9. Kreymann B, et al. Albumin dialysis: effective removal of copper in a patient with fulminant Wilson disease and successful bridging to liver transplantation: a new possibility for the elimination of protein-bound toxins. J Hepatol. 1999;31(6):1080–5.
10. Jhang JS, et al. Therapeutic plasmapheresis as a bridge to liver transplantation in fulminant Wilson disease. J Clin Apher. 2007;22(1):10–4.
11. Rakela J, et al. Fulminant Wilson's disease treated with post-dilution hemofiltration and orthotopic liver transplantation. Gastroenterology. 1986;90(6):2004–7.
12. Grodzicki M, et al. Results of treatment of acute liver failure patients with use of the prometheus FPSA system. Transplant Proc. 2009;41(8):3079–81.
13. Collins KL, et al. Single pass albumin dialysis (SPAD) in fulminant Wilsonian liver failure: a case report. Pediatr Nephrol. 2008;23(6):1013–6.
14. Sen S, et al. Albumin dialysis and molecular adsorbents recirculating system (MARS) for acute Wilson's disease. Liver Transpl. 2002;8(10):962–7.
15. Medici V, et al. Liver transplantation for Wilson's disease: the burden of neurological and psychiatric disorders. Liver Transpl. 2005;11(9):1056–63.
16. Mocchegiani F, et al. Liver transplantation in neurological Wilson's disease: is there indication? A case report. Transplant Proc. 2014;46(7):2360–4.
17. Dhawan A, et al. Wilson's disease in children: 37-year experience and revised King's score for liver transplantation. Liver Transpl. 2005;11(4):441–8.

18. Fischer RT, et al. Prognostic scoring indices in Wilson disease: a case series and cautionary tale. J Pediatr Gastroenterol Nutr. 2011;52(4):466–9.
19. Schilsky ML, Scheinberg IH, Sternlieb I. Liver transplantation for Wilson's disease: indications and outcome. Hepatology. 1994;19(3):583–7.
20. Bax RT, et al. Cerebral manifestation of Wilson's disease successfully treated with liver transplantation. Neurology. 1998;51(3):863–5.
21. Lui CC, et al. Recovery of neurological deficits in a case of Wilson's disease after liver transplantation. Transplant Proc. 1998;30(7):3324–5.
22. Stracciari A, et al. Effect of liver transplantation on neurological manifestations in Wilson disease. Arch Neurol. 2000;57(3):384–6.
23. Walker G, et al. Liver transplant can resolve severe neuropsychiatric manifestations of Wilson disease: a case report. Exp Clin Transplant. 2016.
24. Brewer GJ, Askari F. Transplant livers in Wilson's disease for hepatic, not neurologic, indications. Liver Transpl. 2000;6(5):662–4.
25. Emre S, et al. Orthotopic liver transplantation for Wilson's disease: a single-center experience. Transplantation. 2001;72(7):1232–6.
26. Guarino M, et al. No neurological improvement after liver transplantation for Wilson's disease. Acta Neurol Scand. 1995;92(5):405–8.
27. Kassam N, et al. Liver transplantation for neuropsychiatric Wilson disease. Can J Gastroenterol. 1998;12(1):65–8.
28. Senzolo M, et al. Different neurological outcome of liver transplantation for Wilson's disease in two homozygotic twins. Clin Neurol Neurosurg. 2007;109(1):71–5.
29. Yagci MA, et al. Influence of liver transplantation on neuropsychiatric manifestations of Wilson disease. Transplant Proc. 2015;47(5):1469–73.
30. Ahmad A, Torrazza-Perez E, Schilsky ML. Liver transplantation for Wilson disease. Handb Clin Neurol. 2017;142:193–204.
31. Mogul DB, et al.. Fifteen-year trends in pediatric liver transplants: split, whole deceased, and living donor grafts. J Pediatr. 2018.
32. Schilsky ML. Transplantation for inherited metabolic disorders of the liver. Transplant Proc. 2013;45(2):455–62.

33. Park YK, et al. Auxiliary partial orthotopic living donor liver transplantation in a patient with Wilson's disease: a case report. Transplant Proc. 2008;40(10):3808–9.
34. Haberal M, et al. Auxiliary partial orthotopic living liver transplant for Wilson disease. Exp Clin Transplant. 2017;15(Suppl 1):182–4.
35. Asonuma K, et al. Living related liver transplantation from heterozygote genetic carriers to children with Wilson's disease. Pediatr Transplant. 1999;3(3):201–5.
36. Przybyszewski EM, et al. Durable clinical and immunologic advantage of living donor liver transplantation in children. Transplantation. 2018.
37. Feng S, et al. Complete immunosuppression withdrawal and subsequent allograft function among pediatric recipients of parental living donor liver transplants. JAMA. 2012;307(3):283–93.
38. Cheng F, et al. Outcomes of living-related liver transplantation for Wilson's disease: a single-center experience in China. Transplantation. 2009;87(5):751–7.
39. Yoshitoshi EY, et al. Long-term outcomes for 32 cases of Wilson's disease after living-donor liver transplantation. Transplantation. 2009;87(2):261–7.
40. Miloh T, et al. Immunosuppression in pediatric liver transplant recipients: Unique aspects. Liver Transpl. 2017;23(2):244–56.

Chapter 12
Partnering for Care of Wilson Disease

Mary L. Graper and Michael L. Schilsky

The Physician Team: Diagnosis

Patients often report that their diagnostic journeys to establish a diagnosis of WD involve a complicated process of visiting different healthcare providers. At times patients are misdiagnosed, with the result being a delay in establishing a diagnosis of WD, sometimes for many years [1]. To ensure that your patient being considered for a diagnosis of Wilson disease (WD) receives the best care, assistance from specialists with experience in diagnosing and treating this disorder should be sought. This includes finding an experienced

M. L. Graper (✉)
Wilson Disease Association, New York, NY, USA
e-mail: mary.graper@wilsonsdisease.org

M. L. Schilsky
Division of Digestive Diseases and Transplant and Immunology, Departments of Medicine and Surgery, Yale University, New Haven, CT, USA
e-mail: michael.schilsky@yale.edu

M. L. Schilsky (ed.), *Management of Wilson Disease*, Clinical Gastroenterology, https://doi.org/10.1007/978-3-319-91527-2_12

ophthalmologist who has seen Kayser-Fleischer rings before doing the slit-lamp examination and working with an experienced liver specialist or neurologist who has previously been involved in the diagnostic evaluation of patients with WD. As this disease is relatively rare, most gastroenterologists or neurologists have never seen or have seen only a single patient with WD, and therefore finding liver specialists or movement disorder specialists with the appropriate expertise is important.

If you are unable to travel from your local area to see a WD specialist because of insurance or other issues, here are some tips on how to partner with other specialists who have had experience treating patients with WD:

- Ask prospective physician specialists if they have ever diagnosed or treated WD patients.
- Find out if they are familiar with the current practice guidelines that were published by the American Association for the Study of Liver Disease (AASLD) [2] or by the European Association for the Study of the Liver [3].
- Ask if they are willing to consult with expert Wilson disease treating physicians at one of the WDAs Centers of Excellence (COE) [4].
- Call or e-mail the WDA, and ask if they can refer you to an experienced physician in your geographic area [5]. A partial list of treating physicians is on the WDA website, and another list is maintained internally in the WDAs files.

The Patient's Role

Information about WD should be shared with your patient, and they should be encouraged to continue to read and ask questions to learn how to be good partners in their care. You may have access to other electronic media with medical information about WD; however most patients will not have access to these same advanced medical sites that have peer-reviewed and other vetted publications. There are useful resources on the WDA website that you can refer your patients to. Information on the WDA website is accurate and is reviewed by the Medical Advisory Committee (MAC) of the WDA before it is posted.

Patients should be encouraged to ask for copies of their laboratory results or enroll in programs that allow them access to their laboratory and testing data in electronic medical records. To help them organize their data, we suggest you encourage them to use the Wilson Disease Patient Lab Tracker provided on the WDA website to enter their historic data about disease diagnosis, medications, and lab results. The Tracker lists all of the laboratory tests that are recommended for diagnosis and routine monitoring and helps patients with portability of information that can be used to share with all their providers. The Tracker is organized in a flow sheet format for looking at relevant data for managing patients and adjusting treatments. A sample of the Lab Tracker is included in the Appendix, and a link to the site for download is provided in reference [6] below (Fig. 12.1).

If you are managing your patient's medications for their WD, you will also need to become familiar with what the recommended target result ranges are for good copper control in treated patients. These are discussed in Chap. 6, on Monitoring. The targets for results may differ between treated and untreated patients and for the type of therapy the patient is taking for their WD. These data can be found on the Lab Tracker page on the WDA website [6]. Encourage patients to ask about results that are out of appropriate ranges, and make sure they know when to obtain their next testing. Be aware that reference laboratories report highs or lows based on what they would be in a person without WD, not for a person with WD. Consult with one of our COE directors if the data is concerning or difficult to interpret. These physicians are very experienced in the intricacies of WD treatment and monitoring and can give advice on data interpretation and help with treatment plans.

TREATMENT AND MONITORING OF WILSON DISEASE							
Name: Samuel K. Wilson		Reference	Date:	Date:	Date:	Date:	Date:
Medications	Units	Range	6/18/1998	7/13/1998			
d-Penicillamine	(mg/day)			250 tid**	** qd = once a day		
Pyroxidine (B6)	(mg/day)			50 qd**	bid = twice a day		
Trientine	(mg/day)				tid = 3 x day		
Zinc acetate	(mg/day)				qid = 4 x day		
Zinc (other)	(mg/day)						
Other medications:							
CBC/Platelets							
WBC	K/UL	4.8-10.8	6.4	7.1			
HgB	GM/DL	14.0-18.0	14.1	14.3			
HCT	%	42.0-52.0	41.2	40.9			
Platelets	K/UL	150-400	199				
Liver Function Panel							
Albumin	*Report the units and						
Total bilirubin	normal reference						
Direct bilirubin	values as	your own					
Alkaline phosphatase	lab reports them.						
ALT	U/L	8.0-36	166				
AST	IU/L	13-38	67				
Alphafetoprotein (AFP)							
Coagulation							
INR		0.0-1.1	1				
Prothrombin time	SEC.	22-33	33				
Copper and Zinc Parameters							
Serum copper							
Serum ceruloplasmin	MG/DL	20-40	23				
24 hour urine (copper/volume)	mcg/day	15-50	150	1950			
24 hour urine zinc							
Non-ceruloplasmin copper							
Urinalysis							
Protein							
WBC							
RBC							
Other							
BUN							
Creatinine							
Neurological Symptoms							
Absent	X		X				
Present	X						
Tremors	I NI W						
Speech (dysarthria)	I NI W						
Coordination	I NI W						
Swallowing	I NI W						
Insomnia	I NI W						
Other:							
Psychiatric Symptoms							
Absent	X		X				
Present	X						
Anxiety	I NI W						
Depression	I NI W						
Mood swings	I NI W						
Other:							

FIGURE 12.1 Lab Tracker Image

Advocates

Sometimes patients have difficulty advocating for themselves when they are ill. A social worker can be of great assistance in identifying patients' needs and their available resources. If you have a social worker available to refer patients to, that can often help patients and caregivers with finding the help they may need in a timely fashion (see Chap. 11). If not, patients can hire social workers or other healthcare advocates that may enable them to navigate the complexities of the healthcare system. Many patients may not realize that to share information they may need to sign the proper release of information or records forms, and you may be able to assist them with this process so that they are in compliance with HIPPA regulations [8]. Other patient advocates may include family or friends that can serve as a proxy to effectively communicate the patient's needs to healthcare team members on their behalf [7]. The WDA also aids in patient advocacy. The WDA is not a covered entity as defined by the HIPAA regulations but does everything possible to maintain patient confidentiality while assisting with helping patients and their caregivers obtain the necessary resources for their care.

Wilson Disease Centers of Excellence

What Is a COE?

A Wilson disease Center of Excellence (COE) is designated as such by the WDA and must be affiliated with an academic medical institution. There are currently nine COEs. Six that are located in the United States include Baylor College – Texas Children's Hospital and St. Luke's Hospital in Houston; Northwestern University in Chicago; Seattle Children's Hospital (affiliated with the University of Washington); University of California at Los Angeles; University of Michigan Hospital in Ann Arbor; and Yale University Medical Center in New Haven, CT. Two are located in India at Jaslok Hospital and Research Center in Mumbai and K.E.M in Pune. The ninth and newest COE is located in the United Kingdom at the Royal Surrey Hospital in Guildford [9].

A COE has a healthcare team composed of physicians and other healthcare professionals who are committed to the care of Wilson disease patients. They are well trained in the diagnosis and treatment of WD patients. The director of the COE is responsible for organizing the center and can coordinate referrals and patient care to subspecialists within the center. Often patients require the assistance of more than one specialist, and the ability of these enters to provide multidisciplinary care needed for this disease with the wide range of patient symptoms. There are over 15 specialists at each Center of Excellence. Our COEs, as opposed to most local physicians, diagnose and treat anywhere between 20 and 300 patients annually. When the WDA developed its COE strategy, it had a vision for exceptional patient care. A COE has academic physicians who, in addition to being well informed about WD, are involved in the education of the next generation of physicians, conduct research on WD and publish their work in peer-reviewed journals to advance knowledge among other medical professionals, and provide many of the other services that some patients and families need. The WDA also asks that the institution acts as a counseling resource to patients and other healthcare professionals. They also advise the WDA on medical matters and support various WDA initiatives [10] (Table 12.1).

Why Your Patient Should Visit a COE?

Having your patient treated at a Center of Excellence has many advantages. One of the problems with local care is that you may need to see many different specialists in different locations. The various specialists may not communicate with one another, which can be detrimental to your continuity of care. When you seek treatment at a COE, every healthcare professional and your medical records are all in one place. Many of the centers have regularly scheduled WD clinics when every member of the care team is available to see you on the same day. Appointments can also be arranged as needed outside of scheduled clinic dates. Another advantage is that you may be eligible to participate in any clinical trials

Table 12.1 Members of the healthcare team at a WDA Center of Excellence

Director	Physician in charge of the Wilson disease healthcare team
Hepatologist (adult and pediatric)	An M.D. who has undergone specialized training in the field of gastroenterology and concentrates on treating liver diseases
Neurologist (adult and pediatric)	An M.D. who has undergone specialized training and concentrates on treating disorders of the nervous system
Movement disorders specialist	A neurologist with additional training in the specialty of neurological disorders that affect the speed, quality, and ease of body movements
Ophthalmologist	An M.D. who has specialized training in diagnosing and treating diseases of the eye
Psychiatrist	An M.D. with specialized training in diagnosing and treating psychiatric, behavioral, and emotional disorders
Transplant hepatologist	An M.D. with advanced training in gastroenterology who focuses on the management of advanced liver disease
Fellow	An M.D. who is a board certified specialist pursuing subspecialty training
Resident	An M.D. who has completed medical school and is pursuing advanced training in a medical specialty
R.N. (registered nurse)	Has completed a certified RN program and performs basic medical tasks as instructed by a physician. Often provides educational resources and coordinates your care
Dietician/nutritionist	A specialist who plans diet and nutrition programs for patients with dietary restrictions
Genetic counselor	A healthcare professional who is trained to help families understand genetic disorders

(continued)

Table 12.1 (continued)

Clinical research coordinator (CRC)	A specialized research professional working with and under the direction of the principal investigator (PI) for any clinical trials
Physical therapist (PT)	An expert who is trained to evaluate and treat mobility problems and educate caregivers about how best to provide assistance to the patient
Social worker (see Chap. 11)	A trained professional who assists individuals and families with counseling and by providing resources for financial, employment, disability, and other issues created by a chronic illness
Speech pathologist	An expert trained to evaluate and treat speech, voice, swallowing, and communication problems in patients with WD

that are being conducted to evaluate a new therapy or compare existing therapies. At this writing, there is one new investigational drug in clinical trials at most of our Centers of Excellence and other sites worldwide. Also, just recently launched is the first comprehensive multicenter Wilson Disease Patient Registry. The registry currently has nine patients enrolled and aims to enroll 300 patients over a 5-year period at five institutions in the United States and one in the United Kingdom. The purpose of the registry is to, "help us to understand the epidemiology and natural history of Wilson disease. Our hope is that it will enable us to determine best practices for diagnosis and treatment and support new initiatives for research and patient care" [11, 12]. Once again, this offers patients additional opportunities to participate in research activities.

We took this vision of quality patient care one step further by creating a unique care model called the Wilson Disease Cooperative Network (WDCN) in 2015. The

WDCN is composed of a central site at Yale University, led by Dr. Michael Schilsky, and five other clinical sites headed by investigators who are members of our MAC and/or are COE directors. A liaison from the WDA is also a part of the group. At its inception, the WDCN consisted of five sites in the United States with plans to expand globally. We have already expanded to an additional site in the United Kingdom. "Goals of this network include development of new and better options for the diagnosis, treatment, and monitoring of WD, further study of dosing and efficacy of established treatments, and comparative studies on outcomes of treatment." A key part of this network project is a patient registry, which began enrollment December 2017. A central database and a repository for blood, DNA, and tissue samples of enrolled patients have been established at Yale University. A central laboratory in the United Kingdom has been engaged to do all advanced copper analysis on samples collected from patients enrolled in the registry. Molecular genetic testing will be done at one laboratory at the University of Washington Seattle Children's Hospital under the direction of Dr. Sihoun Hahn, COE director and expert in genetic testing for WD. From these data, we hope to learn more about the current diagnosis and treatment of WD and enable additional translational research and clinical trials [13].

The WDA receives many emails, letters, and phone calls from patients and families throughout the year. Some of them are seeking advice and support. Others are stories of success and praise for the advice and care they are receiving from their healthcare partners. One of the points we hope this chapter was successful in making is that seeking and finding quality medical care is one of the best gifts a patient can receive. The partnership between patient and healthcare team members may change over time and should reflect the potential changing needs of a patient. Being a partner to the process of forming a good care plan and then carrying it out assures that patients optimum health and quality of life while living with their WD.

References

1. Graper ML, Schilsky ML. Patient support groups in the management of Wilson disease. In: Czlonkowska A, Schilsky ML, editors. Handbook of clinical neurology, vol. 142. Amsterdam: Elsevier; 2017. p. 231–40.
2. Roberts EA, Schilsky ML. Diagnosis and treatment of Wilson disease: an update. In: Practice guidelines. American Association for the Study of Wilson disease; 2009. https://www.aasld.org/sites/default/files/guideline_documents/Wilson%20Disease2009.pdf.
3. European Association for the Study of Liver Diseases (EASL) Clinical Practice Guidelines. Management of Wilson's disease. In: Journal of Hepatology. http://www.easl.eu/research/our-contributions/clinical-practice-guidelines/detail/management-of-wilson-s-disease. 2012.
4. The Wilson Disease Association. Centers of Excellence: http://www.wilsonsdisease.org/for-patients-families/centers-of-excellence. 2018.
5. The Wilson Disease Association. http://www.wilsonsdisease.org/. 2018.
6. The Wilson Disease Association. http://www.wilsonsdisease.org/for-patients-families/lab-tracker-copper-calculator. 2018.
7. Graper ML. Wilson disease: maintaining a successful treatment plan. A patient handbook. Milwaukee: Wilson Disease Association; 2008. http://www.wilsonsdisease.org/phocadownload/resources/WD108_Patient_Handbook.pdf. 2018.
8. U.S. Department of Health and Human Services. Health information privacy. Health Insurance Portability and Accountability Act (HIPAA). 1996. https://www.hhs.gov/hipaa/index.html/. 2018.
9. Wilson Disease Centers of Excellence. http://www.wilsonsdisease.org/for-patients-families/centers-of-excellence. 2018.
10. Graper ML, Schilsky ML. Patient support groups in the management of Wilson disease. In: Czlonkowska A, Schilsky ML, editors. Handbook of clinical neurology, vol. 142. Amsterdam: Elsevier; 2017. p. 231–40.
11. Registry for Patients with Wilson Disease. http://www.wilsonsdisease.org/programs-research/patient-registry. 2018.
12. Natural History Study of Wilson Disease. https://clinicaltrials.gov/ct2/show/NCT03334292?cond=Wilson&rank=1 . 2017.
13. Terry CA. The Wilson disease cooperative network (WDCN): a blueprint for the future. In: The copper connection. Wilson disease association, 2015. http://wilsonsdisease.ca/phocadownload/newsletters/Winter20152016Newsletter.pdf. p 5.

Chapter 13
Clinical Research Participation

Ricarda Tomlin

Introduction

Clinical and epidemiological research are the cornerstones to developing better diagnostic, therapeutic, and preventative tools in medicine. Especially in rare diseases such as Wilson disease, collaboration between researchers and patients is key, as there may be multiple trials competing for the same population and it is more challenging to enroll enough participants to lead to meaningful research findings. Some people choose to participate in research because it may provide some personal benefit, and others opt to join to "pay it forward" – recognizing that much of the clinical advancement we currently benefit from relied on those before us who chose to join research efforts.

R. Tomlin, BS
Yale University, School of Medicine, Department of Surgery/Transplant, New Haven, CT, USA
e-mail: ricarda.tomlin@yale.edu

M. L. Schilsky (ed.), *Management of Wilson Disease*, Clinical Gastroenterology, https://doi.org/10.1007/978-3-319-91527-2_13

Participation in research is voluntary and may or may not benefit the individual patient. However, every patient should know about research participation opportunities and receive detailed information to make an informed decision.

Research Types Relevant to Rare Diseases

The United States Congress passed the Orphan Drug Act in 1983 to spur research for rare diseases (those affecting less than 200,000 persons in the USA) by offering incentives to research industry sponsors. This has increased the interest in conducting clinical trials and the rate of development of new treatments for Wilson disease and many other rare diseases.

Clinical trials are interventional studies designed to establish the safety and efficacy of new treatments. Research in rare diseases needs to be conducted with the same scientific rigor and ethical standards as all other clinical research. The gold standard of randomized controlled trials therefore is applied; however slightly modified designs (such as crossover trials or N-of-1 trials where everyone receives the treatment under investigation and the comparison treatment/placebo at some point) might be considered [1]. It is important for researchers to explain the design thoroughly, and patients should be encouraged to ask questions about it. While randomization or use of placebo may raise concerns among potential study participants, the investigator will be able to explain the rationale of the design and safety precautions in place to give all the information needed for patients to make decisions regarding participation.

Patient registries or natural history studies are particularly important in rare diseases as they allow the systematic collection of longitudinal data [2]. Registries are typically non-interventional and collect data and/or specimen from a large pool of patients over a long period of time. While Wilson disease has been treatable for many years now, knowledge gaps in regard to precise diagnosis, best therapy and individualization of treatment, endpoints for treatment, and monitoring of therapy can be addressed with this research tool.

Specimen and Data Storage Provisions

Commonly, samples and data will be *coded* when entered into the repository, meaning the participant's name, medical record number, and other direct identifiers will be replaced with an individual code, and the link between the identity and code will only be accessible to authorized users. This allows the protection of the participants' privacy while maintaining the ability to (1) link data elements with sample analysis results, (2) recontact participants regarding interest in additional future research, and (3) remove samples or data should a patient withdraw consent [3].

Many researchers use the term *de-identified* which we recommend avoiding, since it can be interpreted to either mean coded (unique codes replace direct identifiers) or unidentified/anonymous (meaning no codes are kept with the samples and data).

When investigators seek initial consent from the registry participant, they should provide information regarding whether samples and data will be coded or collected anonymously, who will have access to the samples and data in the future, how access will be controlled, and what type of future research is permitted. It may not always be possible to anticipate all the types of future research to be conducted, so many studies set up oversight to permit or deny access requests to samples and/or data from other researchers [4]. In addition, the participant may be asked to opt for possible contact regarding future research that is not included in the initial consent.

Much of the future in biomedical research rests on genetic and exome analysis, especially in rare diseases. Participants should be aware of what types of genetic testing are planned and be alerted to the potential misuse of genetic information in case of breach of confidentiality. While investigators have safeguards in place and misuse is unlikely, a small risk remains. Discrimination based on genetic information by health insurance companies and employers is illegal since the passing of the Genetic Information Nondiscrimination Act (GINA) in 2008. However, the law does not include provisions against potential discrimination by companies that sell life insurance, disability insurance, or long-term care insurance.

Assuming data and specimen are collected in a coded fashion, participants will maintain the ability to withdraw consent resulting in either destruction of the samples and data or destruction of the link between the study code and identity.

Resources to Find Studies Seeking Participants

In the USA, all clinical trials are required to be registered on clinicaltrials.gov before they open to enrollment, and results will be posted there as well. The website provides a summary of the study, outlines eligibility criteria, and lists study sites and contacts for anyone interested to learn more. The search filter allows to specifically look for studies open to enrollment.

In addition, patient association websites are a great place to look for new studies. For Wilson disease, this association is the *Wilson Disease Association* or WDA, and their website is wilsonsdisease.org.

Rights of Research Participants

The current human subject protection provisions in the USA are based on three guiding ethical principles: respect for persons, beneficence, and justice [5]. Subsequent federal regulation known as 45-CFR-46, or the "Common Rule," [6] translates these principles into specific requirements for a review of all research by an IRB (institutional review board, i.e., an ethics board), requirements for informed consent, and additional protections for vulnerable populations such as pregnant women, children, and prisoners.

The guiding ethical principles are reflected in the elements of informed consent: Before joining any research study, the investigators are responsible for obtaining the potential participants consent in writing or verbally (depending on the complexity and risk stratification of the study). It is important to note that informed consent is not considered a one-time static agreement but an ongoing process. Throughout the course of the study, the participant retains the right to change his or her mind about continued participation, and investigators will update participants about relevant new information or interim findings, especially in regard to safety of an experimental treatment. Table 13.1 outlines the required basic elements of consent, as dictated in the federal regulations [6].

Research participants therefore have the right to receive detailed information about the study before joining and during the course of the study, to be free of coercion to participate, and to expect that their welfare will be protected by the investigators to the best of their abilities.

Table 13.1 Eight basic elements of consent

1	Clear identification of the project as research, an explanation of the purpose of the study and the expected duration of the subject's participation, a description of the procedures, clearly marking those which are experimental
2	Outline of foreseeable risks and discomforts
3	Outline of potential benefits to participants and others
4	Disclosure of alternative procedures or treatments
5	Confidentiality provision
6	Information regarding compensation and economic considerations (i.e., description of whether a sponsor or the participant's insurance will cover the cost of study procedures)
7	Contact information for future questions about the study
8	Emphasis of the voluntary nature of study participation, the ability to refuse participation, or withdrawal from the study without penalty or loss of benefits

Research Participation of Children

Children are an inherently vulnerable population and deserve special protections in research. Not every study may be deemed safe for children to participate in. On the other hand, excluding children from research can lead to knowledge gaps and lack of evidence-based care for children, as they represent a unique population with different needs from adult patients [7].

US regulations (45-CFR-46, subpart D) [6] require investigators to obtain informed consent from parents or guardians, which follows the same guidelines outlined above. In addition to parental consent, researchers will seek assent (affirmative agreement) from children deemed to be capable of providing it (generally starting at the age of 7). This typically involves a developmentally appropriate discussion between the research team and the child, supported by a written assent form outlining the study in age-appropriate language.

Research involving children is typically permitted if the risk is minimal or the anticipated direct benefit to the child justifies the risk. Should the research study involve greater than minimal risk without direct benefit to the child, is it only permissible if it promises to yield vitally important answers in the understanding or treatment of a disorder and will require permission from both parents (unless only one parent has legal custody).

Clinical Research as a Partnership

In any clinical research, the investigators are not only responsible for protecting the rights and welfare of the participants but also for ensuring data quality and reliability. Fulfillment of both goals hinges on establishing good relationships between investigators and subjects [8]. Study participation is not a passive process. Indeed, investigators rely on participants to actively engage during the consent process, provide accurate information, voice concerns, report any adverse reactions, and attend the schedule study visits. For treatment studies, it is important to follow directions for dosing and storage of the study medications, as well as avoiding medications that may be contraindicated. Patients should be advised to consult with the study doctor before starting a new medication while receiving research treatments.

These expectations and responsibilities for participants should be outlined and discussed during the informed consent process, but good communication between the study team and the participants throughout the course of the study is paramount to ensure participants' safety and data integrity.

Sample Flow Chart of a Clinical Trial

Clinical trials typically consist of a number of stages through which participants move. These study components will be outlined in the "Procedures" section of the informed consent document. The components will vary depending on the design of a particular study, so the flow chart below (Fig. 13.1) only serves as an example of the most common stages.

The consent process has already been described earlier in the chapter. The screening phase serves to limit study enrollment to participants who meet the entry criteria outlined in the study protocol. For example, participants with known allergies to study treatments or with comorbidities might be excluded due to safety concerns. The screening phase may just consist of reviewing the participant's medical history, or the study may require certain screening procedures (such as laboratory assessments or an echocardiogram). The results of these procedures may determine eligibility to participate.

If all eligibility criteria have been reviewed and are met, the participant may then be randomly assigned to a study arm or treatment group (see bottom row of Fig. 13.1). Randomization is typically done electronically to avoid any bias. Depending on the design, patients may be able to cross over from one arm to another after a certain amount of time or may be required to stay in the designated arm.

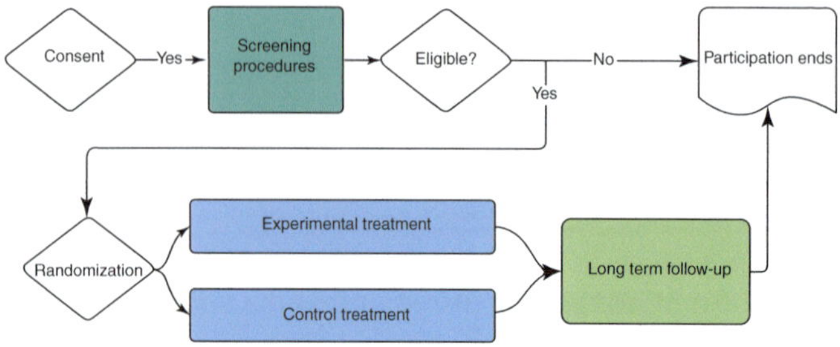

Figure 13.1 Flow chart of a sample clinical trial

Most treatment studies include a follow-up phase to the study which typically consists of fewer study visits or sometimes just phone visits over a long period of time to assess possible long-term side effects and/or long-term efficacy of the treatment.

After the study concludes and all data has been collected and analyzed, study results will be published and accessible to the public via clinicaltrials.gov. Private information about study participants will not be published. Participants may also contact the study team to inquire about results or with other questions.

What Questions Should a PCP/Patient Ask When Considering a Study?

Trusted PCPs may serve as a great resource for patients considering study participation. While the study team may not be able to share the full sponsor protocol with someone outside the study team due to confidentiality constraints, PCPs can review the consent documents with the patient, consult the clinicaltrials.gov listing together, or may agree to speak with the investigator to obtain more information, should patients give their permission.

Here are some questions you may consider asking:

- What is the prior experience with the study medication in humans?
- What are the expected risks and benefits?

- Are there any known drug interactions with other medications?
- Who is sponsoring the study?
- Are there any inclusion or exclusion restrictions that may not permit my patient to participate?
- If there is randomized treatment assignment, what is the ratio between receiving the experimental versus control treatment?
- Is there a placebo arm to the study and how will the patient's condition be treated during this time?
- Is the study blinded, i.e., will the participant and/or the study team know which treatment has been assigned?
- What safety assessments are planned as part of the study?
- Who will cover the cost of the study procedures and treatments?
- How long will the study last? How many visits are anticipated, and how time-consuming will they be?
- Does the study cover travel costs?
- What happens when the study ends? Is there a mechanism for continued access to study medication, if desired?
- How are samples and data kept? For how long? Who will have access?

References

1. Griggs RC, Batshaw M, Dunkle M, et al. Clinical research for rare disease: opportunities, challenges, and solutions. Mol Genet Metab. 2009;96(1):20–6.
2. Richesson R, Vehik K. Patient registries: utility, validity and inference. In: Posada de la Paz M, Groft S, editors. Rare diseases epidemiology. Advances in experimental medicine and biology, vol. 686. Dordrecht: Springer; 2010.
3. Hansson M, Lochmüller H, Riess O, et al. The risk of re-identification versus the need to identify individuals in rare disease research. Eur J Hum Genet. 2016;24:1553–8.
4. Grady C, Eckstein L, Berkman B, et al. Broad consent for research with biological samples: workshop conclusions. Am J Bioeth. 2015;15(9):34–42.

5. National Commission for the Protection of Human Subjects of Biomedical and Behavioral Research. The Belmont report: ethical principles and guidelines for the protection of human subjects of research. Bethesda: The Commission; 1978.
6. Code of Federal Regulations. U.S. Department of Health and Human Services. 2009. https://www.hhs.gov/ohrp/regulations-and-policy/regulations/45-cfr-46/index.html. Accessed 5 Jan 2018.
7. Crane S, Broome M. Understanding ethical issues of research participation from the perspective of participating children and adolescents: a systematic review. Worldviews Evid-Based Nurs. 2017;14(3):200–9.
8. Resnik DB, Ness E. Participants' responsibilities in clinical research. J Med Ethics. 2012;38(12):746–50.

Chapter 14
The Social and Emotional Impact of Wilson Disease on Patients and Families

Lenore Hammers and Mary L. Graper

The diagnosis and related symptoms of Wilson disease create psychological and social challenges for patients, their families, and caregivers. Since most primary care physicians do not have a full-time social worker in their office, it is helpful for physicians to recognize these challenges and to provide direction for patients and their caregivers.

The following checklist is a guide to help understand the common challenges for patients and their families:

L. Hammers (✉)
Yale New Haven Transplantation Center, Liver Transplant Program, New Haven, CT, USA
e-mail: Lenore.Hammers@ynhh.org

M. L. Graper
Wilson Disease Association, New York, NY, USA
e-mail: mary.graper@wilsonsdisease.org

M. L. Schilsky (ed.), *Management of Wilson Disease*, Clinical Gastroenterology, https://doi.org/10.1007/978-3-319-91527-2_14

Emotional

Coping:

Is the patient expressing feelings of sadness? Overwhelmed? Angry outbursts?

Stigma:

Is the patient afraid to tell family/friends/employers about their diagnosis

Social activity vs. isolation:

Is the patient withdrawing from social and family settings?

Interpersonal conflicts:

Does the patient complain of changes or conflict in their closest relationships?

Sexual relationships:

Does the patient report difficulties with sexual desire or performance?

Financial

Income:

Does the patient have adequate income for basic needs (housing, food, utilities)?

Work:

Is the patient able to maintain employment? Are they afraid of being laid off because of the patient's symptoms?

Work resources:

Has the patient inquired about Family and Medical Leave Act (FMLA) to protect his job if he has to miss work for medical reasons? Have they inquired about short-term and long-term disability?

Special accommodations:

Does the patient require special accommodations to maintain his employment?

Insurance:

Does the patient have adequate financial coverage for doctor visits, lab work, and medications? Does the insurance have deductible or co-pays?

Medications:

Can the patient afford his medications? Do they know about patient assistance funds?

Disability:

If the patient is no longer able to work, does he qualify for Social Security Disability, and do they know how to apply?

Caregiver Concerns

Caregiver burnout:

Are the parents, spouse, or caregivers of the patient reporting fatigue, frustration, and anger? Are they finding ways to care for themselves?

Finding additional help:

What is the patient and family network? Does the patient or caregiver know where to look for additional caregiving assistance?

Caregiver employment:

Does the parent, spouse, or caregiver qualify for FMLA to help protect their employment, while they take time to care for the patient?

Finding a patient advocate:

Does the patient or family have an advocate who can help navigate finding support and resources as needed? Are they aware of support groups in their area?

Legal

Power of attorney:

Has the patient appointed a power of attorney to help manage his finances if he is unable?

Healthcare representative:

Has the patient appointed a healthcare representative?

Conservator of person and finances:

If the patient is not competent to appoint a healthcare representative or power of attorney, is there a family member or caregiver who can apply to be conservator?

Legal aid:

Does the patient or caregiver need legal assistance to fight against discrimination or assist in disability claims? Can they afford representation?

Advanced therapies:
Transplant:

Are the Wilson disease symptoms so severe that the patients requires a liver transplant? Does the patient meet the medical and psychological and social requirements to be eligible for a liver transplant?

Long-term care:

If the patient is no longer able to care for himself and the family is also unable to care for him in the home, does he require placement in a facility, either short term or long term? Can he or the family afford it? Do they know how to find appropriate facilities, and are they available?

These concerns will now be explored in more detail.

Emotional and Coping Concerns

Patients with Wilson disease may present with symptoms of emotional distress. Symptoms may range from being mildly withdrawn to more serious symptoms, such as eating too much or too little, withdrawing from family and activities, and not attending to their activities of daily living. In extreme cases, patients may present with symptoms of major depression and suicidal thoughts.

Patients may report feeling burdened by the stigma of a rare and chronic disease. They may be afraid to tell those closest to them they have Wilson disease for fear of being misunderstood or shunned. Since Wilson disease is so rare, their symptoms (such as personality changes, tremors, or even psychotic symptoms) may have been misdiagnosed and misunderstood. Patients may blame themselves for their behavior or experience a disruption in their interpersonal relationships.

One of the best ways physicians can assist their patients in coping with Wilson disease is by providing patients and their caregivers with sufficient information about the disease. Once patients and families understand that some of their behaviors are symptoms of a disease that can be treated the stigma and anger can be mitigated. Having a clear understanding of the nature, progression and treatment of the disease and its symptoms can be empowering.

If the patient is expressing distress over some particular symptoms, just as shaking, confusion, sexual dysfunction, or mental changes, you as the physician can explore ways to treat those symptoms medically and improve their functioning.

When symptoms cannot be completely alleviated, physicians can assist their patients by helping them to reframe their expectations. Patients may express frustrations that they cannot do everything they used to do before they were diagnosed with Wilson disease. A simple expression of empathy can help patients feel heard, less isolated, and thereby relieve some of their stress. Explaining what treatment you can and cannot provide helps the patient understand and accept his limitations. Encourage the patient to optimize the things he is able to do, rather than focusing on those limitations.

If the patient continues to experience ongoing distress, a referral to a therapist or support group may be helpful. A referral to counseling is particularly helpful if the patient exhibits symptoms of major depression or other psychiatric symptoms, such as anxiety and psychosis. A psychiatrist familiar with Wilson disease can be most beneficial, but they are rare. If you are not familiar with local counselors in your area, encourage the patient to contact the mental health referral line located on the back of his insurance card. Patients may also contact the United Way (211) in your state for additional referrals. If you have a social worker or case manager in your office, he may also be able to assist with referrals.

If the patient is a child in school, the parents may contact the school for additional resources. Most schools employ social workers and psychologists who can assist with diagnosing emotional issues, as well as providing support and referrals. Parents may request an interdisciplinary special treatment plan for patients with disabilities, sometimes called a Planning and Placement Team meeting (PPT). The PPT meeting generally consists of teachers, social workers, nurses and others to develop a specific plan to provide appropriate accommodations for the student. If the child cannot manage in a regular school system, the school district may be able to arrange an in-home tutor.

Support groups can be an additional source of encouragement. Attending meetings with other patients and families familiar with Wilson disease can help ease the sense of isolation. Patients and families may also benefit from the wisdom and research of other families who have encountered problems similar to theirs. If a patient does not have access to a local support group, the Wilson Disease Association (WDA) has an official Facebook page on which information is posted and updated on a regular basis. The WDA also has a closed Facebook page (19), administered by two WDA administrators, specifically for young people with Wilson disease, so they may share their concerns privately. An Internet-based healthcare support community called Inspire offers an avenue for patients and caregivers to provide mutual support to other families coping with Wilson disease. Member names on the Inspire website are anonymous unless individuals choose to identify themselves.

If you have concerns that a patient is so severely depressed he may be a danger to himself, don't be afraid to ask directly if he is feeling hopeless or suicidal. If a patient expresses any suicidal ideation, someone should stay with the patient while someone else in the office calls 911 to bring the patient to the emergency room for assessment. Alternatively, if you are in a clinic attached to a hospital, and the patient is willing, a staff or family member may walk the patient into the emergency room and wait with the patient until they are evaluated.

Financial Concerns

One of the biggest concerns for patients facing Wilson disease, similar to other chronic diseases, is financial stress. As the symptoms progress, patients may find it difficult to maintain employment. Even if patients are able to work, they may find the cost of co-pays, coinsurance and medication costs overwhelming. Patients may face the additional stress of time out of work, leading to additional lost income. If a parent or spouse must also take time off of work, the financial strain on the family will only increase.

A patient may be concerned he will be terminated from his employment due to workdays missed for medical reasons. Encourage the patient to contact his human resource department, if there is one at his place of employment. Some companies will offer Family and Medical Leave Act (FMLA), which protects the worker's employment if they need to be out of work for their own illness or that of a close family member. The patient's human resource department will generally supply paperwork for the patient's physician to complete, indicating the nature of the illness, the impact on the patient's employment, and the anticipated time out of work. The patient may apply for intermittent leave (i.e., half a day out of work once or twice a week) or continuous leave (when a patient will be hospitalized or otherwise unable to work for an extended period). The patient should be aware that his employer is not required to pay him for the time off and will generally require the patient to use his allotted sick leave before using FMLA benefits.

Some employers offer short-term and long-term disability benefits, which would allow the patient to collect income while he is out of work. The benefits vary, but generally short-term disability applies to patients who will be out of work for less than 6 months and will pay a portion of the patient's salary (60–80%). If the patient will be out of work longer than the short-term disability term (usually more than 6 months), he may be eligible for long-term disability. Patients may also inquire whether or not their paid time off can be used to supplement their short-term or long-term disability income.

If it becomes clear the patient will not be able to return to their previous employment due to the physical or mental limitations of Wilson disease, the patient could request reasonable accommodations to help him perform his job or request a different type of work within the company, if possible, which he is able to perform.

There may come a time when your patient is physically or mentally unable to work in any capacity. Some states offer temporary disability benefits, most do not. If the patient is expected to be unable to work for more than a year, he may be eligible for Social Security Disability (SSD) income benefits. Patients can apply for SSD benefits by calling or making an appointment at the local Social Security office or by applying online at SSA.org. The Social Security office will obtain releases of information from the patient for all their medical providers and will request medical records directly from the providers. Some Social Security offices may also require a statement from a physician. The patient should be informed that the application process can be complicated and lengthy. The patient may choose to hire a lawyer to help with their disability claim. Most lawyers will not charge a fee upfront but will take a portion of the disability claim once it is granted. Patients may also contact Allsup.com (17) for assistance. Allsup will assess the patient's eligibility for Social Security benefits and assist with the application process. They also do not charge a fee upfront but will take a portion of the benefits if the claim is successful.

The patient's insurance can have an impact on the patient's out-of-pocket expenses. Patients' out-of-pocket costs will vary, depending on whether they have commercial insurance, state insurance (Medicaid), or federal insurance (Medicare).

If the patient has commercial insurance, he can call the customer service line listed on the back of the insurance card to inquire about co-pays and deductible costs for office visits, blood tests, and hospitalizations. If the patient is married, he can inquire if the spouse's insurance can offer better coverage and if he can be added to the spouse's coverage. The patient can also ask which doctors are in network with their particular insurance, because they will generally pay a smaller co-pay for doctors who are in network. If the patient loses his employment, he may be eligible for COBRA insurance, allowing him to maintain his employer's insurance for some period after the employment ends. Unfortunately, those COBRA premiums are usually expensive. The patient may want to investigate whether their state offers access health insurance policies or if they would qualify for state insurance (Medicaid).

State insurance (Medicaid) generally offers zero to low premiums or co-pays, but patients need to meet income guidelines. Patients should contact their Department of Social Services to determine if they are eligible for any state insurance programs.

Patients are eligible to receive Medicare if they have reached retirement age, have been on dialysis for 3 months, or have been receiving Social Security Disability benefits for 2 years. Patients will usually pay premium payments for Medicare B and their prescription plans (Medicare D). The State Department of Social Services may offer Medicare Savings Plans to offset the cost of these premiums for qualified patients.

Some patients may have difficulty paying for their medications due to high co-pays or because the insurance does not authorize it, forcing the patient to pay the entire cost out of pocket. You, as the physician, may contact the insurance company to explain why a medication is needed, and the insurance company may agree to pay for it. Otherwise, you might consider an alternative medication which is less expensive. Walmart has a program offering $4 co-pays for some medications. A list of those medications can be found online. The patient may also want to contact the manufacturer of the medication. The manufacturer may offer a patient assistance program or direct the patient to available grants to pay for the medication. The patient may also look for the medication on the website needymeds.com (10). In some cases, the manufacturer will offer a co-pay card to reduce the cost of the medication, which can be downloaded off the website and provided to their pharmacy. The local pharmacist may be an additional resource for finding ways to lower the cost of the medication.

If your patient is having significant difficulties meeting their basic needs, such as rent, food, or housing, the patient may contact the Department of Social Services in their area or the United Way (infoline.org or 211) for additional community resources.

Caregiver Concerns

Coping with Wilson disease can take a toll not only on the patient but also on the families and caregivers. Caregivers may be coping with the patient's mood swings and tremors and in some cases providing almost constant care. In any case, being a caregiver can be exhausting.

As previously mentioned, caregivers will benefit from learning as much as possible about Wilson disease. As is the case with the patient, having a clear understanding of the symptoms, progression, and treatment options can lessen the anxiety of the unknown. As a physician, explaining the needs of the patient and the caregiver's role will allow the caregivers to plan and give them a sense of control.

Ideally, there will be more than one person caring for the patient. As a physician, you may want to ask about the family network. Are there other available family members in the area? Are the caregivers part of a local church, congregation, or social network from which they can draw emotional support or practical help? Encourage as many caregivers as possible in the family network to be involved and educated about Wilson disease. Having an expanded network can help decrease the sense of isolation for caregivers and help prevent misunderstanding about the patient's behavior and prognosis. Caregivers may be reluctant to involve other friends or family members, not wishing to be a burden on anyone else. Sometimes simply acknowledging that caretaking is exhausting and giving the primary caregiver permission to look after themselves are a great comfort.

If the caregiving role requires missing work, the caregiver can also explore whether or not their employer offers FMLA benefits to care for immediate family members.

If the patient is a child and the caregiver is the child's parent, the school nurse or social worker may be able to assist with finding additional resources in the community. If the child is considered disabled, the parents can apply for Social Security Income (SSI).

Having an advocate, such as a social worker or case manager, to help navigate all these various systems can be very helpful, but they can be hard to find. If the patient is hospitalized, he can request to meet with a social worker. However, even if the social worker provides resources, the worker is often unavailable for additional assistance once the patient is discharged from the hospital. In some hospital-based clinics, social workers may be available both in the hospital and clinic and thereby provide continuity.

If not, caregivers can look for alternative advocates. The advocate may be a friend or relative who is familiar with some of the systems or has the time to learn about them. It may be someone they meet in a Wilson disease support group. If no specific support group is available (and they usually aren't), finding a support group for other chronic diseases may be useful. Although most Wilson disease patients are young, caregivers may find some help or referrals from the Agency on Aging, where social workers are familiar with resources for caregivers. The Department of Social Services may offer grants or other assistance for long-term care in the home. The Alliance of Professional Health Advocates (18) offers a directory of patient advocates that a patient may hire for a fee.

Legal Concerns

Some patients with Wilson disease may have episodes in which they are not mentally competent to manage their own health and financial concerns. These episodes may be temporary or may extend for longer periods of time. During these episodes, someone else (preferably a close family member) will need to make medical and financial decisions for the patient.

Having the patient appoint a healthcare representative is the easiest way to ensure there is someone to make medical decisions on behalf of the patient if the patient is temporarily unable to do so.

A patient may also want to complete a living will, or advanced directives, to indicate which types of treatment the patient would or would not want to have at the end of their lives. If neither a healthcare representative nor a living will is completed, and medical or end-of-life decisions needed to be made, the medical team would turn to the patient's legal next of kin to be the decision-maker. The chain of legal next of kin runs from spouse to oldest adult child, to parent, and to oldest sibling. Healthcare representative and living will forms can be obtained from any lawyer's office or may be available online. Some states require a healthcare representative form be notarized, some do not.

A power of attorney (POA) document allows someone else to make financial decisions for a patient if he is not competent to make his own decisions. Patients should be careful about whom they appoint as power of attorney, since the POA has the legal ability to withdraw money from a bank, buy property and conduct business on behalf of the patient, unless the patient expressly limits those abilities. The patient can designate whether or not the power of attorney document will remain valid if the patient becomes incapacitated. Most states will require a notary and two witnesses to sign a power of attorney form.

The healthcare representative, living will and power of attorney documents must be completed when the patient is mentally competent. If the patient is not mentally capable of completing the forms and requires someone to make decisions for him, a family member will need to file for conservator of person and estate. The family will need an evaluation from a physician or psychiatrist, attesting that the patient is not capable of making his own decisions. The application is then submitted to the probate court, and a judge will schedule a hearing to decide if the patient requires a conservator or not. If the patient does require a conservator, most judges prefer to appoint a close family member. If no family member is available, he may appoint someone in the community (usually a lawyer or social worker). A conservator may be appointed either temporarily or permanently, depending on the projected period of the patient's incapacity. A temporary conservator can generally be appointed more quickly and will only be appointed if there is evidence that the patient will suffer irreparable harm (physical or financial) if there is no conservator. There is usually a cost to apply for conservator, but if the family cannot afford the fee they can request the charge be waived. If someone is appointed as temporary conservator and the patient still requires a conservator after the temporary date expires, the conservator can apply for an extension or to be appointed the permanent conservator. The conservator document can be revoked by the probate court if the patient's mental status improves and no longer requires a conservator.

A patient may enlist a lawyer to complete a will or to assist in any other legal matters. If a patient cannot afford legal fees, he may contact the United Way to inquire if he qualifies for legal aid.

Patients may pursue legal assistance if they feel they are being discriminated against at their place of employment. The Americans with Disabilities Act makes it unlawful for an employer to fire or discriminate against an employee with a medical or mental disability, provided they are qualified and able to perform the essential requirements of the job. If a patient believes his employer is discriminating against him because of the symptoms of Wilson disease, he should contact the Equal Employment Opportunity Commission. He may also choose to seek legal representation or consult with the union (if there is one).

Advanced Therapies

Liver Transplant

As Wilson disease progresses, a physician may determine that the patient requires a liver transplant.

Not every state has a liver transplant program. If you, as the physician, have determined that a liver transplant is the best option for your patient you can consult the United Network of Organ Sharing (UNOS) website. There you will find the nearest liver transplant program, as well as how the programs compare with other programs. You may want to explore issues such as proximity to the patient to the transplant center, which transplant programs are covered by the patient's insurance, the number of transplants each center performs, and the rate of favorable outcomes.

To be eligible for a liver transplant, a patient will need to meet requirements for both the medical indications for a transplant and the psychological and social guidelines of the transplant center.

All transplant programs are required to have a social worker available to assess the patient's readiness for transplant and to help provide resources and referrals to address any identified barriers to transplant. Some programs also offer psychiatrists and psychologists.

Although programs vary, there are several social and psychological parameters the patient will need to meet to be eligible for transplant at most centers. At a minimum, the patient will need to demonstrate that he has a stable environment in which to recover from a liver transplant. He will need to have at least one support person who is willing to encourage him to take medications and be willing to bring him to follow up appointments. If the patient has a mental health history, the center will require the patient be in treatment or demonstrate that the symptoms will not hinder the patient's ability to take medications and follow through on treatment recommendations. If the patient has severe cognitive deficits as a result of Wilson disease, the center will evaluate whether or not those symptoms can be reversed after a liver transplant. The center will evaluate the patient's history of adherence to medical appointments and to taking medications. If the patient has a substance abuse history, most centers will require the patient to demonstrate 6 months of continuous sobriety, along with a commitment and plan to maintain sobriety after transplant. Most centers will require the patient to complete some type of substance abuse treatment prior to listing. The patient will also need to demonstrate that he has adequate insurance and financial resources to pay for the transplant and lifelong medications. Most centers will not accept a patient who is not a documented citizen, or who is in the United States illegally.

Long-Term Care

Some patients may become so debilitated that they cannot be safely cared for in the home with only family support. In some states, the Department of Social Services will offer grants to provide extensive services at home, although sometimes the patient will need to be in a facility for some period of time before those services are offered. Patients may require either short-term or long-term care in a nursing facility. Unfortunately, most nursing facilities are oriented toward elderly patients, which can be frustrating for younger Wilson disease patients. Patients and their families may ask the discharge planners at the local hospital (usually a nurse or social worker) if they know of any facilities who serve younger patients.

Most insurance policies have limited coverage for nursing facilities. A patient may need to exhaust their assets to qualify for state assistance to pay for long-term care. Patients and their families may investigate facilities in their area, but usually the easiest way to place a patient in long-term care is through the hospital.

Appendix

The following check list is a guide to common challenges for patients with Wilson disease and families:

Emotional

Yes ☐ No ☐ Coping: *Is the patient expressing feelings of sadness? Overwhelmed? Angry outbursts?*
Yes ☐ No ☐ Stigma: *Is the patient afraid to tell family, friends, or employers about their diagnosis?*
Yes ☐ No ☐ Social activity vs. isolation: *Is the patient withdrawing from social and family settings?*
Yes ☐ No ☐ Interpersonal conflicts: *Does the patient complain of changes or conflict in their closest relationships?*
Yes ☐ No ☐ Sexual relationships: *Does the patient report difficulties with sexual desire or performance?*

Financial

Yes ☐ No ☐ Income: *Does the patient have adequate income for basic needs (housing, food, heat)*
Yes ☐ No ☐ Work: *Is the patient able to maintain employment? Are they afraid of being laid off because of their symptoms?*
Yes ☐ No ☐ Work resources: *Has the patient inquired about Family and Medical Leave Act (FMLA) to protect his job if he has to miss work for medical reasons? Have they inquired about short-term and long- term disability?*
Yes ☐ No ☐ Special accommodations: *Does the patient require special accommodations to maintain his employment?*
Yes ☐ No ☐ Insurance: *Does the patient have adequate financial coverage for doctor visits, lab work, and medications? Does the insurance have a deductible or co-pays?*
Yes ☐ No ☐ Disability: *If the patient is no longer able to work, does he qualify for Social Security Disability, and does he know how to apply?*

Caregiver Concerns

Yes ☐ No ☐ Caregiver burnout: *Are the parents, spouse, or caregivers of the patient reporting fatigue, frustration and anger? Are they able to care for themselves?*
Yes ☐ No ☐ Finding additional help: *What is the patient and family network? Does the patient or caregiver know where to look for additional caregiving assistance?*
Yes ☐ No ☐ Caregiver employment: *Does the parent, spouse, or caregiver qualify for FMLA to help protect their employment, while they take time to care for the patient?*
Yes ☐ No ☐ Finding a patient advocate: *Does the patient or family have an advocate who can help navigate finding support and resources as needed? Are they aware of support groups in their area?*

Legal

Yes ☐ No ☐ Power of attorney: *Has the patient appointed a power of attorney to help manage his finances if he is unable?*
Yes ☐ No ☐ Healthcare representative: *Has the patient appointed a healthcare representative?*
Yes ☐ No ☐ Conservator of person and finances: *If the patient is not competent to appoint a healthcare representative or power of attorney, is there a family member or caregiver who can apply to be conservator?*
Yes ☐ No ☐ Legal aid: *Does the patient or caregiver need legal assistance to fight against discrimination or assist in disability claims? Can they afford representation?*

Advanced Therapies

Yes ☐ No ☐ Transplant: *Are the Wilson disease symptoms so severe that the patient requires a liver transplant? Does the patient meet the medical and psychosocial requirements to be eligible for a liver transplant?*
Yes ☐ No ☐ Long-term care: *If the patient is no longer able to care for himself and the family is also unable to care for him in the home, does he require placement in a facility, either short -term or long -term? Can they afford it? Do they know how to find appropriate facilities, and are they available?*

Online Patient Resources

1. Wilsons Disease Association: wilsonsdisease.org
2. Family Caregiver Alliance: caregiver.org
3. National Center on Caregiving: caregiver.org/national-center-caregiving
4. Family Voices (for children's healthcare concerns): familyvoices.org
5. The Caring Action Network (CAN): caregiveraction.org
6. HealingWell.com
7. Rare Disease United Foundation: rarediseaseunited.org

8. American Liver Foundation: liverfoundation.org
9. needymeds.com
10. Patient Access Network (PAN): panfoundation.org/.
11. HealthWell Foundation: healthwellfoundation.org
12. Children's Organ Transplant Association: cota.org
13. National Foundation for Transplants: transplants.org
14. Help Hope Live: helphopelive.org
15. Allsup.com
16. The Alliance of Professional Health Advocates: aphadvocates.org/directory
17. Wilson Disease Association Facebook page: facebook.com/wilsondiseaseassociation
18. Wilson Disease Association group on Inspire: inspire.com/groups/Wilson-disease-association

Index

M. L. Schilsky (ed.), *Management of Wilson Disease*, Clinical Gastroenterology, https://doi.org/10.1007/978-3-319-91527-2

MIX
Papier aus verantwortungsvollen Quellen
Paper from responsible sources
FSC® C105338

If you have any concerns about our products,
you can contact us on
ProductSafety@springernature.com

In case Publisher is established outside the EU,
the EU authorized representative is:
Springer Nature Customer Service Center GmbH
Europaplatz 3, 69115 Heidelberg, Germany

Printed by Libri Plureos GmbH
in Hamburg, Germany